2010

D0251047

Babushka's Beauty Secrets

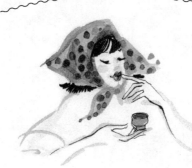

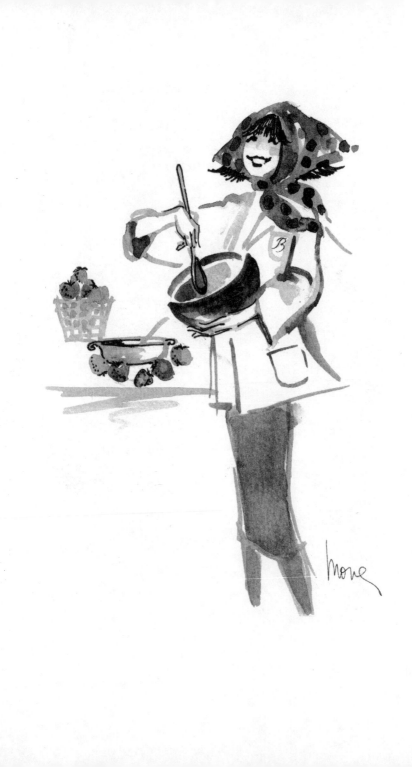

Babushka's Beauty Secrets

Old World Tips for a Glamorous New You

RAISA RUDER AND SUSAN CAMPOS

Illustrations by Mona Shafer Edwards

WELLNESS CENTRAL

NEW YORK   BOSTON

Wellness Central
Hachette Book Group
237 Park Avenue
New York, NY 10017
www.HachetteBookGroup.com

Wellness Central is an imprint of Grand Central Publishing.
The Wellness Central name and logo are trademarks of
Hachette Book Group, Inc.

Printed in the United States of America
Book design by Fearn Cutler de Vicq

First Edition: June 2010
10 9 8 7 6 5 4 3 2 1

Library of Congress Cataloging-in-Publication Data
Ruder, Raisa.
Babushka's beauty secrets : old world tips for a glamorous new you / Raisa
    Ruder and Susan Campos. — 1st ed.
      p. cm.
Includes index.
ISBN 978-0-446-55586-9
1. Beauty, Personal.   2. Feminine beauty (Aesthetics)   3. Beauty shops.
    I. Campos, Susan.   II. Title.
HQ1219.R83 2010
646.7'042—dc22

                              2009030438

Contents

~~~~~~~~~~~~~~~~~~

Contents

Acknowledgments

This book never would have been written if it weren't for my fantastic clients, who are open to trying new masks and creams. Thank goodness for Molly Lyons, who believed in this project. Diana Baroni has been incredible in the entire process. We are very appreciative.

A special thanks to Mona Edwards and Lauren Tejeda, who are so creative. And to our parents, families, and friends who are always open to trying new lotions and potions. Thanks to Ben, Eugene, and Alex. And this book wouldn't be possible if it weren't for my babushka. She would have loved it!

Babushka's Beauty Index

Babushka's Beauty Secrets

Chapter One

My Babushka's Beauty Secrets

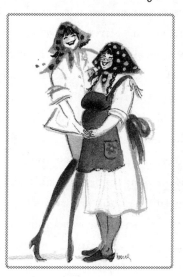

NAME: Raisa Ruder

HAILS FROM: Ukraine and Moscow

OCCUPATION: Esthetician (with leanings toward the
Green Party)

CURRENTLY RESIDES IN: Los Angeles, California

AGE: Once you become a Hollywood citizen, there's no
need to reveal your true age.

*A*bove are my vital statistics. For the past fifteen
years, Los Angeles has been my home, where I work
as an esthetician. In the Ukraine, my grandmother (or

as we say back home, my babushka) taught me everything about being a natural esthetician. By taking items such as fruit, milk, herbs, teas, and other ingredients, we'd whip up fabulous facials. Rather than use creams and lotions laced with preservatives, we preferred applying natural products — it saved our skin and it saved us money!

Who knew several decades later the recipes my grandmother concocted would become all the rage in Hollywood. In a city always on the cutting edge of beauty, it seems ironic to be applying my babushka's age-old recipes on some of the most famous faces in Tinseltown. While I love doing oxygen facials, power peels, and lasers, my true passion is brewing up beauty and saving money doing it. The recipes in this book are (mostly) all-natural remedies I use to maintain Hollywood's youthful glow — from exfoliating scrubs to vitamin C serums to hair treatments. I've mixed up my favorite concoctions — some of my grandmother's original Ukrainian recipes — as well as others I've doctored up since moving to the United States. Here's my motto: Why spend hundreds at a department store makeup counter when you can create it yourself for a fraction of the price? After whipping up and trying these recipes, I promise you'll feel like you've spent hundreds! Just as the weekly magazines show us how to get celebrity clothing for less, *Babushka's Beauty Secrets* creates glowing skin for under $5.

My grandmother didn't believe in being wasteful. She saved everything. My clients love hearing stories about how my grandmother was virtually a pack rat. Her house was so neat and clean but she couldn't help saving every item or finding another purpose for it.

You see, strictly out of necessity we were making the equivalent of modern-day products without the fancy names, pretty packaging, and preservatives. Decades later, I still believe my babushka's beauty remedies can go head to head with any department store brands. Rather than pay $250 for expensive labels, my grandmother's recipes were fresh, fantastic, and inexpensive! The box below reveals what we were brewing in our tiny village years ago and how it prices out against department store products today.

Department store vitamin C serum	= $250 vs.	Babushka's olive oil, orange, and lemon serum	= $1.95
Revitalash	= over $100 vs.	Babushka's castor oil concoction	= less than $1.00
Eye moisturizer	= $150 vs.	Babushka's apple/honey remedy	= $0.50
Quick dry for nails	= $28.59 vs.	Babushka's sunflower oil	= $0.25
Deep hair conditioner	= $90 vs.	Babushka's mayonnaise mask	= $2.00
Alpha hydroxy cream	= $78 vs.	Babushka's strawberry mask	= $3.50

The satisfaction of knowing you saved hundreds by using products that are just as good (if not better) and preservative free in most cases = PRICELESS!

The beauty business brings in $40 billion a year. Most of it is wrapped up in pretty packaging. This book proves that a bigger price tag isn't necessarily better—homemade products can produce the same results without bursting your bank account. Many dermatologists even agree that expensive brands aren't always better. In fact, many of the products they tout are heavily diluted by the time they reach department store shelves.

Big beauty companies know the importance of ingredients such as retinol (vitamin A), antioxidants, vitamin C, and alpha hydroxy acids. These are buzzwords commanding big money for beauty in a bottle. But I'm going to show you how there are quick, inexpensive ways to get a boost without buying expensive brands. Below are three of the hottest ingredients on the market today and different ways to mimic their effects on the skin naturally:

1. **Alpha Hydroxy Acids.** Alpha hydroxy acids (AHA) are the hottest ingredients to hit the beauty business. They are found in a number of expensive beauty lines and are perfect for sloughing off dead skin. But before you go spending hundreds of dollars, just know that foods such as pineapples, strawberries, apples, and even milk are overflowing with AHAs. So why not go directly to the source? Many of the recipes in this book are filled with AHAs. When applied to the skin, they penetrate the

upper layer to peel off dry skin and welcome new healthy cells. If you pamper your skin constantly with AHAs, it will begin to regularly exfoliate—as it did when you were in your teens.

2. Vitamin C. Vitamin C serums are big in beauty as well—in some cases selling for hundreds of dollars for a few ounces. There is nothing better for a beautiful glow than a little serum on the skin. But it's so easy to duplicate the magic in a bottle. This book has tons of easy recipes filled with vitamin C. Do you have lemons, limes, oranges, tomatoes, or raspberries in your home? You don't need them all; one will do. Those are just a few of the natural products with heavy doses of vitamin C. No need to pay hundreds of dollars when it's already in your home.

3. Antioxidants. Antioxidants are a brilliant way to preserve younger-looking skin, fight free radical damage, and promote overall health. With all the recent talk about antioxidants, why not embrace fruits such as blueberries, blackberries, raspberries, and pomegranates. Beauty companies put a small amount of these fruits (or green tea) in their products and tout them as high in antioxidants. Can they help reduce aging when used topically? I say yes, they can! But know you can do it for less! Why not go directly to the source and save money at the same time.

⌒ ⌒ BABUSHKA'S WAY ⌒ ⌒

My grandmother did go directly to the source for everything. Without all the research, she innately knew it
worked. This is a woman who ate raw garlic every day.
In addition to believing it was a natural antibiotic, she
loved what it did for the skin. Sure her breath took a hit,
but she thought it was well worth it. My grandmother was
so resourceful she made her own breath mints to combat
the odor.

She had a natural remedy for everything. It seemed
as if she never left the kitchen. If she wasn't cooking a
meal, she was brewing up beauty. You see, my babushka's
recipes are ingrained in my mind after watching my
mother and grandmother create masks ever since I was
a little girl back in the Ukraine. Without even knowing
it, my babushka was a kind of visionary in the world of
green beauty. When I was young, we were making masks
every day—cooking up preservative-free potions, recycling, reusing, and doing it all on a bare-bones budget.
Even as a young teen I truly idolized my babushka. She
was like a rock star among certain women in our small
Ukrainian village. With all the information stored in
her head, she was a brilliant esthetician. She could whip
up a natural bromide for everything from acne to puffy
eyes to blackheads. I'd watch as she'd rattle off age-old
beauty recipes the way Julia Child used to throw together
a soufflé.

Beets (a favorite in the Ukraine) would be the main

ingredient to naturally color the lips of a brunette, while blondes might get a concoction with carrots. She didn't have set fees for facials. Instead women would pay whatever they could afford. It was an honor system and it didn't matter to my babushka because she was passionate about natural beauty.

As a teenager, my grandmother began getting interested in these natural recipes, but she didn't really hit her stride until the age of thirty-two. In her small Ukrainian town, they'd use herbs and natural remedies to heal cuts and bring down fevers. Over the years she began to manipulate and reformulate recipes. People couldn't believe the results! She began building a name and a very modest business.

As the matriarch of our family, she believed every woman should be a good cook. It was incredible to watch her maneuver around a hot stove, whipping up masks and potions. Slowly her friends began spreading the word and my babushka's house became a hot spot in our small town.

Women entered our tiny, low-ceilinged home, and my grandmother would throw together one of her famous natural remedies. Imagine three generations of women (my grandmother, my mother, and myself) running a makeshift spa from a tiny house perched at the end of a long dirt road.

A coterie of women would literally stand in line waiting to see my babushka. The walls inside the tiny kitchen (the heart of our home) were lined with rows and rows of shelves—filled with everything from special salt to rare Russian herbs. And the refrigerator was no different—it was packed with every kind of fruit and vegetable we could get our hands on. Like any patriotic Ukrainian (remember, we were once part of Russia), we were always sure to stock two items: potatoes and vodka.

Despite bitter cold weather, women would trek through the snow to get an appointment with my babushka. In the beginning, it was a few people every couple days, but by the time I turned ten, there were up to fifty women of all ages coming through our home each week. It was incredibly rewarding to see how the salves from my grandmother's humble kitchen brought smiles to the faces of so many women in our town. One treatment and they became converts.

In addition to slathering potions on a client, my babushka would dish out advice on everything from saving one's marriage to getting a man. Whether a problem of the skin, or one of the heart, she wasn't afraid to tackle it.

Clad in a full-length black skirt (her pockets filled with herbs), a traditional Ukrainian shirt, and a shawl wrapped around her shoulders, she'd putter around the kitchen with purpose. Oh, I almost forgot the most important part. She would always wear a scarf around her head (the term *babushka*, referring to a folded kerchief that is tied around the hair, originates from the fact that older Russian women customarily wore the traditional head wrap).

My grandmother was truly passionate about her products. The first thing my babushka did each morning was boil hot water and make a huge pitcher of black tea with a dash of cognac (those tea leaves would later be used for a facial she would whip up for a client since nothing went to waste). Then she'd fire up the stove and start cooking her concoctions.

✳ BABUSHKA'S ADVICE ✳

Not only did my babushka empower women by creating beauty on the outside, but she also taught them to take control of their personal relationships. When they were having difficulties with their husbands, she was famous for saying, "A woman is the neck and a man is the head. And the head can never move without the neck!" Ironically, I heard the same line years later in the film *My Big Fat Greek Wedding*. I thought, "Greek women get it, too."

Known for her enthusiasm and energy, my grandmother was a real character. She would always create a fun environment. Just as you might see in a restaurant, my babushka would even offer up a daily special using different kinds of food we had around. For instance, if we had an excess of potatoes (it's such a Russian thing), we'd whip up something special with them. (You can't believe what a potato will do for bags under the eyes!)

We made complicated masks without blenders or measuring cups. Because my babushka knew all her recipes by memory, she never used traditional measuring devices. She would literally bend down to table level and eyeball the ingredients. She'd pour a little bit of this or a dash of that—then stir, smash, and mix everything up to perfection!

When I came to the United States and people would ask for recipes, I'd literally say things like a "handful of flour" or a "squirt of buttermilk." Babushka's measurements worked something like this:

One dash = $\frac{1}{16}$ teaspoon

One pinch = $\frac{1}{8}$ teaspoon

A sprinkle = 1 teaspoon

A squirt = 1 tablespoon

A handful = $\frac{1}{4}$–$\frac{1}{2}$ cup (depending on the size of your hands—my babushka's were huge!)

A double handful (cup both hands together)

= $\frac{3}{4}$–1 cup

Don't worry: For the purposes of this book, proper measurements are included in each and every recipe. While I still don't use measuring cups, I do love modern household conveniences such as blenders and food processors. We did everything by hand! My grandmother would have loved a blender.

Recycling was big, too! We'd often use the skin of a potato, the shell of an egg, or the seed of a grape rather than throw them away. There was no waste when mixing up our recipes. Decades later and thousands of miles away, those strict guidelines are still a major part of my practice. When I was fifteen, we had the rare luxury of getting a pumpkin. I was about to throw away the seeds when my grandmother shot me a dramatic look. I stopped in my tracks. It was like throwing out diamonds and pearls. She took them out of my hands and explained how pumpkin seeds have so many nutrients. "This is where it all starts," she explained. She smashed them up and we used them in a body scrub.

Those days, working side by side with my mother and grandmother, were some of the happiest and most creative times of my life. Back then, my grandmother was my mentor and I became her eager apprentice. By the time I was thirteen, she trusted me to diagnose a problem and make up a mask on my own.

We all had our favorite ingredients and would experiment with different masks. While my mother and I loved working with fruits such as berries and papaya to create various masks, my grandmother was old school and preferred potatoes. We would try out different concoctions on one another and fine-tune the end product. They taught me how to whip up a natural remedy for just about any skin problem.

Importing these recipes to America was never part of my grandmother's master plan. Nor was it really mine. She'd be proud to see some of her original recipes in this book, and wouldn't mind the fact I've doctored up others

✳ BABUSHKA'S TOP FIVE INGREDIENTS ✳

1. **Potatoes**: I think it was because they were so available. However, they do serve multiple purposes.

2. **Vodka**: Again, it was so available and a national treasure. Just know it is the best preservative.

3. **Milk**: She loved the vitamins in milk and how it acted as a sort of bleaching agent for the skin. I always think how she'd love those "Got Milk?" commercials.

4. **Olive oil**: Olive oil was a luxury for my grandmother. If it hadn't been so expensive back then, we would have used it daily. Sunflower oil became the substitute. The winters were so brutal that oil became a daily ingredient in all of her recipes. Throughout Europe, women love olive oil for the skin.

5. **Eggs**: Since she used every part of an egg, my babushka really got every penny out of it—from the shell to the yolk.

since moving to the States. She'd be proud of my new creations as well. Most are all natural, and in only about 10 percent of the recipes do I permit store-bought creams or canned goods strictly for the sake of saving time (but you'll still save money, too). I often think my babushka would suffer sticker shock to see the prices of lotions and masks today.

She'd be outraged to see the prices consumers are paying in the name of beauty. Simply put, pure products are more effective than those laced with tons of preservatives.

You get better results and it's much healthier for the skin.

Like my grandmother, I became a passionate natural esthetician—moving to Moscow to attend school and work. In 1994, I brought my family to Los Angeles. I remember coming to California and working in a Beverly Hills salon doing eyebrows, power peels, and oxygen facials. The results were fantastic but I couldn't get my grandmother's recipes out of my head.

On the weekends my Russian friends would come over and we'd experiment with new masks. Suddenly there were new ingredients available to me. I was like a kid in a candy store since the grocery stores in the Ukraine didn't even remotely resemble markets in the United States.

In the beginning, I'd just do my babushka's recipes on the weekends since the thought of trying them on a client was a bit intimidating. Then one day I got up the nerve to try a natural recipe on a Beverly Hills client. When she picked up the mirror and saw her glowing reflection, she grabbed my hand and asked, "What did you put on my skin?" A few days later, I broke out the natural remedies on more clients. Word spread quickly through Hollywood.

At my salon, masks are mixed up in minutes. With this book, you can do the same in the privacy of your own home. Simple ingredients found in most American kitchens can change your skin. Just load up the grocery cart with fruits, vegetables, and dairy products and welcome to the beauty business. My clients love how leftovers

✳ WHAT WOMEN WANT ✳

*T*he longer I work in L.A., the more I am convinced women share the same concerns. In my practice the most common complaints are:

1. Cellulite

2. Wrinkles

3. Acne

4. Weight

5. Dry skin

can shave five years off their faces, or how recycling ingredients can give their skin a calcium shine, or how one simple ingredient (no prep work) can literally save them time and money and create glowing skin!

There is no reason to spend excessively on beauty products. Rather than blow $100 on some expensive mask, save it for a purchase you really need. The recipes in *Babushka's Beauty Secrets* are inexpensive (most are under $5), natural, and effective! In this book, I offer up mixtures for everything from getting rid of age spots to banishing acne. You'll learn that bananas aren't just good to eat but brilliant for diminishing crow's-feet and fine lines. If you want to have baby-soft feet, just add a little sugar or salt to your body lotion. Both are fantastic for removing dead skin from the feet and even bringing up those stubborn ingrown hairs.

There's even a chapter dedicated to leftover recipes. Maybe your husband only drank half a beer the night before. Don't throw it out! There's nothing better than flat beer to give the hair a little lift. I also believe there are certain recipes that are good for specific age groups. Chapter 12 is dedicated to the issues of the different decades of life. Maybe the problem is acne in the twenties and dry skin in the sixties. What about when you have only a couple of minutes and can't put too much energy into prep work? Chapter 13, one of my favorites, introduces you to "one-ingredient wonders." With one ingredient, you can give your skin a little glow! You won't believe the results!

A client told me how she was having breakfast at a restaurant recently and put several one-ingredient wonders into effect outside the home. There was a slice of orange on her plate, and she began rubbing the pulp on her skin. She also asked for a side of avocado, and when she didn't eat it all, she smashed it up and applied it to her skin in the restaurant! Not to be outdone, her friend (also a client) did the same! It can be done anywhere if you're brave.

I don't expect women to be so brazen in a restaurant but I know all of our homes are filled with beauty products we don't even realize exist. There is nothing better than the pleasure of pampering the body and face. Imagine being able to enjoy that feeling in your own home— without the big bill. So put on a mask, sip a glass of wine, and watch one of your favorite television shows. Let's get started!

Chapter Two

Let's Get Started

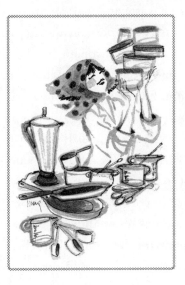

This chapter is all about having the proper tools and stocking the key ingredients. Trust me, it's all very easy. You don't need to be a good cook. My method is far from difficult. It's just a new way of looking at beauty. To make it most efficient, be sure to have key tools and ingredients on hand. Once everything is in place, it's a pretty easy routine to follow.

The results will hook you in! I have a client who'd have those days where she'd wake up and despise her skin. Upon looking in the mirror, she'd run off to the depart-ment store and ask for the latest miracle cream. But in the end, none of the creams or masks lived up to her expectations. It was a waste of time, energy, and money.

I tell this story because some people initially balk at preparing their own masks and creams. But think of the endless hours we waste at department store counters and you'll realize it isn't so time-consuming.

My babushka believed women (in the Ukraine) spent most of their time cooking in the kitchen or getting ready in the bathroom. Funny enough, those are the best rooms to use for mixing up masks. It's also the place to discover key utensils you've got stashed. It could save you a trip to the store. Why leave those tools inside cabinets when they can be part of the beautifying process?

Items such as cotton swabs, old toothbrushes, and combs can come in quite handy. At home, I simply apply masks with my fingers but some of my clients prefer using brushes or cotton balls. In addition, there are certain tools one must have to whip up the various recipes. So before getting started, let's do a checklist.

MUST-HAVE TOOLS

1. Blender. You will be using a blender for 80 percent of the recipes. A food processor will work just as well. Sometimes I even find myself mixing up the easy ones using the little machine that grinds my morning coffee beans.

2. Cotton balls or swabs. You will definitely use these regularly but I try as much as possible to use washcloths so we don't create more waste. Unfortunately, sometimes cotton balls and swabs work better than washcloths because they can get into the hard-to-reach crevices on the face, hands, and feet.

3. Washcloths. There are plenty of opportunities to use washcloths. Always have them handy!

4. Butter knife (for the perfectionist). I have clients who prefer using a butter knife to spread the mask just right. It does really help avoid a mess when applying around the hairline.

5. Measuring cups. Although my babushka loved eyeballing ingredients when creating her beauty recipes, these are modern times and I suggest getting the measurements correct.

6. Measuring spoons. Again, my babushka used a dash here and a sprinkle there, but it's important to get the measurements right!

7. Saucepans. Usually we'll just need a small or a medium saucepan for these recipes.

8. Bowls. Small- or medium-sized bowls will do unless you're having a spa party, and then you may want to double or triple the recipes.

9. Empty bottles. Reuse old bottles that contained shampoo, conditioner, lotion, etc. These can store the different potions and lotions.

10. Plastic containers (even if it isn't always politically correct). Although I try to be as green as possible, sometimes it doesn't work in every situation. Having different-sized containers on hand definitely helps.

MUST-HAVE INGREDIENTS

Preparation

You always need to stock up on the staples. Mine include everything from green tea to milk—essential ingredients called for in a number of my recipes. By having ten basic items, you will be creating your own personal spa at the drop of a hat. Remember, *Babushka's Beauty Secrets* is about achieving the most glamorous look from your own kitchen.

Find a place in your cupboard to store a few products. It will be helpful if you can make a little room in the refrigerator as well. I have a client who dedicates the top shelf of her pantry to beauty ingredients. The refrigerator reflects the same. Her family knows it's a hands-off area.

In addition to key ingredients, there are little tricks to making one's skin look fabulous. For instance, I may ask you to rinse with milk or mineral water (once in a while) rather than from the tap. Maybe it doesn't sound like a big deal, but it makes a huge difference. Milk is a good source of calcium. Not to mention, milk acts as a sort of bleach on the skin. Though tap water is fine at times, it can be a bit harsh on the skin with certain treatments.

My babushka used to say, "If you want to have the skin of a baby, wash with milk." I completely agree. After all, a baby is drinking milk all day long and getting all that good calcium. Who can beat baby skin!

My babushka's recipes didn't have scientific research behind them since she was formulating recipes by mixing her common sense with her knowledge of certain herbs and different kinds of foods. Decades later, her information was right on target with what's going on with cosmetic companies today—from antioxidants to vitamin C. But the real beauty is how she managed to do this all on a budget.

The following is my top ten list of ingredients you should stock in your kitchen. Trust me, they will come in handy.

Top Ten Ingredients

1. **Mineral magic.** No need to wash the face every day with mineral water, but after a good mask, it can be nourishing for the skin. Sometimes tap water is too harsh on the skin, and with certain masks, rinsing with mineral water is the perfect way to get the pure benefits. Mineral water can be like a micromassage for the skin and is great to use before applying moisturizer. It's particularly good in the harsh winter months. It was a favorite for us back in the Ukraine, where the weather could be brutal and beat up our skin. Even in the States, clients can really see the difference when

they rinse with mineral water. It definitely gives skin a nice glow!

2. Vitamin E-xcellent. Vitamin E is a critical part of the antiaging machine. There are many good brands in capsule form at places such as Whole Foods (just look on the back of the bottle to make sure it isn't diluted with anything else). You will find vitamin E oil in most cosmetics, but there's a slight problem—most cosmetic companies add other ingredients and additives, which leaves it only about 20 percent pure.

I know that vitamin E placed directly on the skin can work wonders. As women, we have to deal with everything from wrinkles to stretch marks. Other than olive oil, there doesn't seem to be anything better for preventing stretch marks than vitamin E. As soon as any client gets pregnant, I immediately put her on a combo of vitamin E and olive oil. Not to mention, vitamin E is great on the face for everything from preventing wrinkles to repairing sun damage after a heavy burn. Some believe it even works to repair the skin and prevents scarring after a deep cut.

3. All-over olive oil. Olive oil comes in different varieties. I recommend using extra virgin since it's considered the best and least processed (extra virgin is the oil from the first "pressing" of the olive). Olive oil is great for the face and the body. Sophia Loren credits virgin olive oil baths with keeping her skin youthful. The ancient Romans were famous for bathing in olive oil. Of course, my grandmother was a fan and liked to use it in many recipes—from removing makeup to moisturizing the skin. Back then it was a bit too expensive, though, so we mainly used sunflower oil. Now, I'm obsessed with olive oil! I keep it in my shower and use it on my skin every day.

4. Green teatime. Any box of green tea bags will do. There is so much information out there right now about how green tea is a great antiaging product. It is thought to be one of the most potent antioxidants known to mankind. Antioxidants are those agents that counteract the effects of free radicals. Highly aware of these benefits, beauty companies are scrambling to put green tea in just about every product line. But there's no reason to use it in a diluted form when there's access to the real thing. I truly believe in drinking green tea and using it on the face as well. My grandmother loved a variety of different teas. As more studies reveal the positive effects of green tea, I find myself using it in my practice more and more.

5. Honey. Honey is great for so many things. It contains vitamins, minerals, and amino acids. I love to use it in masks for the face. This wonderful beauty aid nourishes the hair, too. You can put in your tea as well! Honey makes a dramatic difference on the skin. It's also an antibacterial and a fantastic moisturizer. My grandmother used to put a thin layer of honey on her face and then place a layer of buttermilk over it. After twenty minutes she'd wash it off and put on olive oil, followed by her nightly moisturizer. She felt the honey kept the moisture in her face. After a honey-buttermilk mask, she'd wake up the next day and rave about how "Honey is magical."

6. Milk does a face good. Milk will help moisturize the skin while at the same time tighten wrinkles and refine pores. You may be wondering how to wash the skin with milk without wasting it. There are plenty of ways. Pour less than a ¼ cup in a small bowl and apply using a cotton ball. I use milk a lot in this book because it's good for the face and the entire body. My grandmother used to believe in taking an exotic bath in milk (I'm not talking about filling up the entire tub with milk—just adding a cup of it in the bath). She considered milk a very mild bleach and extremely good for the complexion. My clients rave about it now, but they were a little skeptical in the beginning.

7. Bathe in buttermilk. Buttermilk is nothing short of amazing! Rinse the skin with this and you'll see a big difference! It changes the skin. Buttermilk is loaded with live bacteria and puts the good stuff back in your body, especially after a round of antibiotics. In addition, buttermilk is a brilliant cleanser and very kind to the skin. I will often suggest rinsing your skin in buttermilk after doing a particular mask. My grandmother thought buttermilk was one of the best products ever! Cultured buttermilk was not generally something we'd just go buy at the store. Instead, we'd go to a friend's farm and prepare sour milk from raw milk.

8. Flour power. This is good to have to correct recipes that may be a bit watery. One day you may be mixing a mask and feel it's too thick or too thin. When it's too thin, you can add a little flour since we don't like to waste anything. Or if it's too thick, adding a little water can make the consistency just right. I remember when my grandmother was making a special soufflé for a client who had pretty severe brown spots. Since we didn't have a blender back then, she was stirring it up but it was just too thick and lumpy. She added a whole egg and then it became much too watery. Instinctively she added a tablespoon of flour and the texture was just right. I wondered whether the client would like it. Funny enough, she wasn't aware of the drama going on in the kitchen and raved about how much she loved that particular mask. You can use white or wheat flour. I prefer white flour because it serves as a good bleaching agent.

9. Almond oil. This oil is great for the complexion and it's inexpensive. Since the oil is easily absorbed into the skin, it isn't greasy. Almond oil is in a number of cosmetic lines and is wonderful for moisturizing the skin. This ingredient is called for in many of my recipes, so try to have it on hand. Sometimes you can replace it with olive oil. However, with certain remedies it's better to use what's called for in the actual recipe. Almond oil is also great on its own as a moisturizer when the skin is really dry.

10. **Vodka.** I've saved the best for last! Vodka was not just a popular drink in our home, it was a national treasure. *Vodka* in Russian means "little water" or "dear water," and it's a profound part of my business since it's the ultimate preservative. After all, according to legend, it was invented in 1503 by Kremlin monks. They used it as an antiseptic before drinking it (so you see it has always served multiple purposes). For the purpose of this book, it's used mainly as a preservative since it will triple the life of the final product. Rather than throwing out a leftover mask after a week, adding a little vodka makes it last a month! To do so, simply add a dash of vodka before putting it in Tupperware or reusing an old shampoo bottle. Red wine works as well (maybe I'm biased, but I think vodka is better). My clients are often surprised to find out that vodka can really preserve a mask.

My grandmother (like many others) used to say, "Russians may not have tons of grapes, but we do have lots of grain."

In Russia and the Ukraine we take our vodka very seriously! So much so there's a museum dedicated to vodka in Moscow. This clear drink has become synonymous with Russia and it's a vital part of the culture and history of the country. Not to be outdone, the Ukraine followed with its own vodka museum but, in a one-upmanship sort of way, put the museum inside a distillery. Wait until you see all the other uses for this liquid gold.

Did you know vodka can . . .

   1. Remove a bandage. Pulling off a bandage can hurt. Ouch! Pour vodka on the bandage and it dissolves the adhesive.

   2. Clean your glasses. The vodka will clean the glass and kill any bacteria.

   3. Give your razor nine lives. Pour some vodka into a cup and soak your razor blade after shaving. Vodka will prevent the blade from getting rusty and clear any buildup of bacteria.

   4. Work as an astringent. Using a cotton ball, apply vodka (with water) to your face as an astringent to cleanse the skin and tighten pores.

   5. Remove excess glue left behind by a sticker (great for people with children). Rub the leftover glue with a vodka-soaked washcloth.

6. Soothe a sore throat. Add a tablespoon of vodka to a glass of warm water and gargle. The alcohol helps numb the sore throat.

7. Ease the pain from a toothache. Take a shot of vodka when you have a toothache. Swish it around your mouth and let it soak into your gums.

8. Get rid of foot odor. Simply pour out a shot of vodka for each foot and rub it all over. No more funky odor.

9. Remove lipstick stains. Put vodka on a washcloth and rub the stained area. Then put the piece of clothing in the washing machine or send it to the dry cleaner.

10. Help you get over a boyfriend. Pour a shot of vodka in a glass over ice and add club soda (low-calorie). Or add grapefruit juice, orange juice, or tonic. *Na zdorovie!* (Translation: Cheers, salud!)

We have all become accustomed to instant gratification. It's tough to be patient since many of us are used to walking into a doctor's office and having our wrinkles simply disappear.

This book isn't about that. Sure, many of the recipes will have immediate results like plumping up the lips or giving the skin an instant glow, but don't go in with such expectations. The best results will show up in six weeks to three months. If you are diligent about doing the recipes on a regular basis, you won't believe the dramatic change in your skin!

Just be disciplined about it and you'll reap the benefits. I remember one client who came to me weekly for masks after seeing how wonderful her best friend's skin looked in just a few months with me. On her fourth visit, she said, "These masks are wonderful but I'm not seeing the same results as my friend." I pointed out how her friend had been coming to me for a few months and she needed to be patient. At the end of the second month, she was overwhelmed by the transformation in her skin.

I have divided this book into over a dozen different chapters. They deal with everything from creating the perfect spa to recycling beauty to buffing the body. Each chapter has recipes that will surprise you, and that I guarantee will change your skin. Nothing makes me prouder than to see my babushka's recipes receive such a warm reception from new generations of women. Enjoy!

Chapter Three

Create a Fab Five-Star Spa

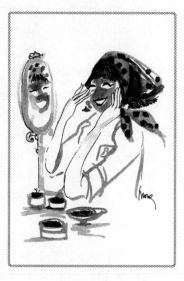

*W*hat if you could hang out in a five-star spa that was actually affordable? Imagine the staff offering good music, top chick flicks, appointments any time of the day or night, and the perfect product line complete with scents tailor-made just for you! Does it sound too good to be true? It's not. Not only does this spa exist, but it's actually in your own home.

Going back to the days of our makeshift spa (at my grandmother's house), I didn't completely appreciate the amazing atmosphere my babushka created. You see, my babushka (like other older women in the Ukraine) was famous for feeding anyone who visited her home. She loved to cook and wouldn't allow anyone to leave without a full stomach. So she offered food and facials.

It was such a relaxing and festive atmosphere. Women would come to decompress from the stresses going on in their daily lives. Our home was a refuge from the daily grind.

Today we all have stress in our lives and there's nothing better than a little pampering to wash away a difficult day—especially when it's inexpensive and guilt-free. You can enjoy a home spa on your own, with a mate, or with a group of women. In Los Angeles, I do parties where women cook up dinner and masks. Trust me, it's fun and addictive!

HOW TO SET UP YOUR HOME SPA

It's actually quite easy. Make sure all your guests bring a comfy robe (or sweats) and slippers. Don't forget the weeklies and the fashion magazines to catch up on all that frivolous reading. Just relax and forget about everything else going on in your life.

Step 1. Set the Mood

Designate a small area where everyone can gather, eat, and hang out. Offer up everything from signature cocktails to fantastic finger foods! Definitely have some mellow music playing in the background to set the mood.

Don't forget to . . .

* Light unscented candles to create a tranquil and peaceful feeling. I recommend unscented so you don't offend your guests.

* Buy some lavender spray. My favorite brand is called Aura Cacia Aromatherapy (available at Whole Foods or at various sites online).

* Provide water with flavored ice cubes. Don't throw away the peels from the lemons, oranges, and limes! These can be incorporated into various recipes. You can also use them to make flavor-infused ice cubes! Simply grate up the peel from a lemon, a lime, or an orange and place the shavings inside an ice cube tray. Fill with water, but leave a little room to top off each cube with a few drops of juice from each fruit. These ice cubes offer just a hint of flavor for a lighter taste and the colorful peels look beautiful inside a glass of water.

* Take the extra juice from the lemon, lime, or orange and put it into a sink filled with hot water. Let a number of washcloths soak inside for 20 minutes and then squeeze out the excess water. Now just throw them in the dryer and you'll have scented towels.

* Find the esthetician. Either hire a professional or decide who will take on that role. I've seen many teenage daughters happily volunteer. Or maybe the hostess?

✳ Give massages. You can hire a massage therapist for your party, but if you're on a budget, simply take turns giving one another massages, facials, and pedicures.

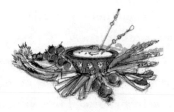

✦ Step 2. Create the Menu

Food

Some of my party favorites include:

FINGER FOODS ~ These include small sandwiches, vegetable platters, etc.

SMOOTHIES ~ Some of the same ingredients will go into your masks.

SWEETS ~ How about strawberries and oranges dipped in chocolate sauce?

Drinks

COCKTAILS ~ My signature spa cocktail is made of vodka and pomegranate juice (since it's a great antioxidant), or club soda with lime for reduced calories. Or maybe you prefer strawberry margaritas?

✳ FRUIT KEBABS ✳

I mpress your guests with this fresh twist on the traditional kebab! Set aside grapes and whole strawberries without the stems while you slice up fruit such as bananas, cantaloupe, honeydew, and pineapple (it's important that the pieces are thick enough so they don't fall apart while you're putting the kebabs together).

Once all your fruit is sliced up, stick wooden skewers through the pieces. Get creative and stack the fruit on the skewers in different combinations and patterns (but make sure to leave enough space at the bottom so your guests can pick them up). Then, put all the fruit kebabs out

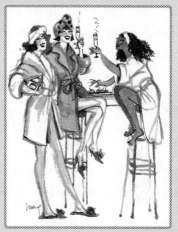

on a tray—or even arrange them in a vase to make a colorful centerpiece. Offer small bowls of yogurt as dipping sauce and let your guests enjoy this fun and healthy treat!

Place green grapes (cut in half) in a separate bowl so your guests can apply them directly to the skin. Just rub the green grape juice near crow's-feet. Grapes are a good source for plumping skin and reducing the look of wrinkles.

COFFEE AND TEA ~ Tea, coffee, and milk can all be used for your masks as well. Don't throw away used tea bags since they are fantastic for reducing puffiness around the eyes.

Decide on Which Recipes You Want to Make

I think a vitamin C infusion after a mask is a big crowd-pleaser. You can make the mask go with the meal and drinks. For instance, if you're serving strawberry margaritas, then definitely make some kind of strawberry mask.

Step 3. Put Together a Playlist

Remember, the point of throwing a home spa party is getting everyone together to relax and have a fun evening! This isn't an evening out on the town, so the music you play should be mellow. Keep it simple and relaxing.

Step 4. Set Up the Facial Area

Decide which area of the house you'd like to transform. Maybe it's the kitchen counter or the bathroom? Just know there are a few things you'll need. Definitely pick a location close to a sink to rinse off masks and an area to store those scented towels. I think it's best to also have a mirror nearby so everyone can get the whole "wow" factor once they wash off the masks. Speaking of those towels, don't forget to pull them out of the dryer at the

✴ CAFÉ DEL MAR ✴

They call it chill-out music on the island of Ibiza. If you want to try something a little different on the music scene, check out Café Del Mar music. Café Del Mar is actually a bar located in San Antonio, Ibiza, that produces ideal music for a five-star spa.

It's a popular summer tourist destination, known for its fantastic view of the local sunset.

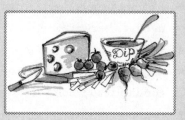

The Café Del Mar releases compilation albums with tracks selected by the bar's own DJs. The music selection is mellow and reflects the mood one would get watching the sunset or relaxing in a spa!

last minute for your guests. What's more luxurious than a warm towel on your skin after a facial!

Spa for One

Sometimes I like to do spas with groups; other times it's just about relaxing on my own. I refer to these evenings as my solo spa nights.

So the next time you just need a little quiet time, try hitting the solo spa.

Solo spa checklist:

✳ **Bubble bath.** I have a recipe in the next chapter that you will love!

✳ **Loofah.** I love doing a little body scrub with a loofah.

✳ **Towel.** Take it out of the warm dryer just before getting started.

✳ **Lotion.** Remember, the bath can be drying, so you'll need it afterward.

✳ **Candles.** Light them to set the mood.

✳ **A good book or magazine.** You'll want something good to read when you soak in the bath.

✳ **A glass of wine or a cup of tea.** It will help you relax.

✳ **Turn off everything from your home phone to your cell.** You won't be able to truly relax when your phone is ringing off the hook.

✳ **Relax and enjoy!**

Before you begin, decide which type of bath you'd like to take. The next chapter offers a number of great recipes that will leave you feeling like a new person! My babushka would always say, "A warm bath washes away a tough day." Creating your own home spa can be invigorating for the body and soul. But I can't indulge in a home spa without soaking in a nice bath, too! One of my favorite recipes is the milk bath in the next chapter. You'll also love throwing together your own bath salts. It's easier than you think!

Chapter Four

Rest and Relaxation

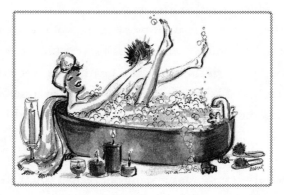

 here's nothing better than a warm bath! This chapter
is dedicated to a little R&R with different recipes for
milk soaks, bubble baths, and even for creating your own
scented lotions. No need to buy those expensive, drying,
perfumed bath salts when you can whip them up in the
privacy of your home. Before getting in a bath, I always
fill the room with steam from the shower to add a little
moisture to the skin. Sometimes, I'll even throw a little eucalyptus essential oil on the floor of the shower to
create a healthy scented steam.

In Eastern Europe, we have always known baths and

steams can be very good for one's health. In Russia, people are fond of something called the *banya*. These are basically steam rooms that have been used for centuries by the Russians. Baths are wonderfully healing and can dramatically reduce stress. Ingredients such as Epsom salts are fantastic for detoxification by bringing out the toxins in the skin. My babushka thought baths were the ultimate in luxury. Although she lived in a small home, she created five-star baths! Whenever we were stressed or upset, she'd make up the perfect bubble bath with a beautiful home-made scent. Whenever I'd step into the bath, I'd feel like royalty, and suddenly my troubles seemed to vanish. This chapter offers up some amazing old recipes you'll love! So pick a recipe, draw the water, and relax!

Babushka's Bubble Bath

Try a little pampering with a luxurious bubble bath. We loved those evenings when my babushka would draw us a warm bath. To this day there is nothing more relaxing for me than a bubble bath, and I still consider them a special treat.

Total time:
5 minutes

INGREDIENTS

    1 cup extra-virgin olive oil

    ¼ cup honey

    ½ cup liquid soap (Most of the big chains carry a
        number of unscented soaps.)

    1 tablespoon essential oil

Put the oil into a blender and slowly add the remaining ingredients. Blend on high for 1 minute. Pour the mixture into a reusable bottle and put on the lid. Shake well before using. Now add some to the bath!

Milk Bath

There's an old legend about how Cleopatra loved to bathe in milk. For centuries, women have indulged in milk baths because of the soothing and moisturizing effects. Here is a milk bath that's quite easy to make using ingredients from the kitchen. It isn't Cleopatra's exact recipe, but it's as close as it could get.

INGREDIENTS

> 1 cup powdered milk
> ½ cup Epsom salts
> ¾ tablespoon baking soda
> 1 teaspoon cornstarch
> A few drops essential oil

Total time:
5 minutes

Simply mix all the ingredients together in a medium-sized bowl. Add to your bathwater and enjoy!

✳ ROYAL MILK ✳

Babushkas are famous for sharing incredible stories. My grandmother would tell us about how Cleopatra bathed in milk—an expensive and rich skin treatment back in those days. We never realized why milk worked, only that it did! Now we know that the lactic acid in milk is an alpha hydroxy, which helps get rid of dead skin while moisturizing at the same time.

Lovely Lavender Bath

These days many people prefer goat's milk to regular milk. So here's another luxurious recipe that takes advantage of this other kind of milk that people with allergies will adore. Remember milk has a form of AHA that is fantastic for the skin. Not only does it nourish the skin but it will help with exfoliation.

Total time:
5 minutes

INGREDIENTS

1 cup goat's milk

1 tablespoon extra-virgin olive oil

A few drops lavender

Mix the goat's milk, olive oil, and lavender together in a medium-sized bowl and stir with a metal spoon since a wooden spoon will soak up all the fragrance. Then place the mixture in a container of your choice, shake it up, and add some to your bath. When you're done, store any unused portion in the refrigerator. You'll love the feel of your skin while bathing in this mixture.

Babushka's Beauty Tip:

Goat's milk is all the rage in Hollywood. Many actresses believe in giving their small children goat's milk rather than whole cow's milk. Women love putting it on their faces as well, since it's known to be extremely gentle on the skin.

Rosewood Scrub

My babushka believed certain scents could change your mood. Lavender is known to be very calming. Have you ever noticed how it's always a popular scent in spas? There's a reason for that. This scrub will be both relaxing and therapeutic for the tootsies. So relax—you've had a long day and deserve to get pampered in the privacy of your own home.

INGREDIENTS

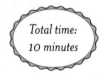

Total time:
10 minutes

1 cup brown sugar

¼ cup almond oil

½ teaspoon vitamin E

2 drops rosewood essential oil

3 drops lavender essential oil

Mix all the ingredients together in a medium bowl and stir well. Apply the mixture to your feet and gently rub. It will be so soothing and relaxing! This is one of those rare times I love mixing two scents together.

Tea Up

Instead of bath time—it's teatime. Actually, it's both. Tea is one of the most soothing things for the soul. My grandmother drank black tea every day, all day. Since coming to the States, I've switched to chamomile. It helps me sleep, quiets my nerves, and just makes me feel comfy. This recipe calls for tea in the bath, and believe me, it will be relaxing. There is nothing more relaxing than lounging in a little chamomile tea.

INGREDIENTS

Total time: 10 minutes

½ cup sea or Epsom salt

2 tablespoons chamomile flowers
(Get them from the tea bags.)

¼ cup dried rosemary

½ cup dried flower petals (Get them from old
flowers in the house.)

2 tablespoons dried lemon or orange peel
(Simply dry out some orange or lemon peel
in the sun.)

Combine all the ingredients in a medium bowl. Mix together, pour into the bath, get a good book, and relax. I like to do this before getting into bed. My grandmother believed baths were the most natural way to relax the body before bedtime. And we all know chamomile is an excellent natural sleeping aid.

Whipped Cream and Oats

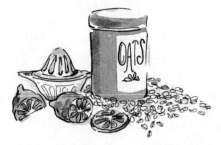

If you've had a stressful day, try this recipe. It's perfect for a solo spa day. Take a little chamomile tea, your favorite gossip magazine, and

put on a mask while you slip into a nice warm bath. This is a calming remedy. You may actually forget what you were so worried about.

INGREDIENTS

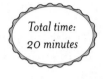

Total time:
20 minutes

>   2 tablespoons finely ground
>   powdered oats
>   1 tablespoon honey
>   2 tablespoons warm whipped cream
>   2 drops tea tree oil

Combine the whipped cream and honey in a small bowl and stir well. Next, add powdered oats and stir. Add tea tree oil and stir again until it's a smooth blend. Apply to your face for 15 minutes, rinse, and follow up with moisturizer. Store any unused mixture in the refrigerator to keep it fresh. Add a dash of vodka to preserve it for a few extra weeks.

Aromatherapy Bath Salts

Bath salts are so therapeutic and relaxing. Shockingly, making your own aromatherapy salts isn't too difficult. You'll take pride in doing this, avoid harmful perfumes, and save money. What could be better? They make great gifts, look beautiful in the bathroom, and will make you feel as if you're on vacation. Light some candles, throw on some mellow music, and read a good book while you bathe in luxury.

INGREDIENTS

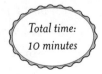

Total time:
10 minutes

>   3 cups Epsom salt
>   1 cup baking soda
>   1 cup sea salt

3 drops of any fragrance (e.g., lavender, tea tree oil)
A few drops of the fragrance from the recipe above
or a store-bought essential oil

Use a large spoon (although I use my hands) to combine the ingredients. Next, you'll want to begin mixing the fragrance oils with your salts. Add a couple drops at a time (so as not to make it too fragrant), and then add a few more. Finding the balance of being able to smell it, but not making it too strong, can be a bit tricky. So take your time. Remember you'll be adding these to your bathwater, which will dilute the scent quite a bit.

Orange Glow

My grandmother loved the smells of everything from flowers to oranges. She never wore perfume but did find ways to make beautiful scents out of natural products. These days there's so much controversy about fragrances that are put into laundry products, cleaning supplies, and bath soaps. With complaints of certain scents wreaking havoc on chemically sensitive people, there is a call for more and more products to be unscented. Now you can control the scent. This next recipe will teach you to make your own essential oil. I use it to spice up moisturizer or bath salts. It's truly amazing and doesn't contain any harmful chemicals.

INGREDIENTS

    Peels from 4 oranges
        (or lemons or limes)
    2 cups olive oil

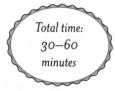

Total time:
30–60
minutes

Put the white part of the peels (do not use the outermost skin itself) into a Crock-Pot on low heat. Throw in the oil. You can also put it on the stove on very low heat (make sure to cover it). Let it brew for about 30 minutes to an hour and you won't believe the results.

Babushka's Beauty Tip:

In the summer months try making the same recipe but add fresh flowers from the garden. Just as a flower is blooming, pick it and place the oil in the jar, then add a tablespoon of the flower petals and stir. Cover the jar tightly and leave it for 48 hours in a sunny windowsill, or place the jar outside in the sun. Shake it up every 12 to 24 hours.

Get a bowl and a piece of muslin. Open up the jar and pour the mixture over the bowl with the muslin in place as a strainer. Squeeze the flowers to extract as much liquid as you can into the jar and you're good to go.

Scent of a Woman

Rather than spend tons of money buying scented lotion, why not make your own? Simply get some unscented lotion and add your own mixture of scents. Personally, I love Eucerin lotion since it's unscented and a fantastic moisturizer. Not to mention, it's recommended by many dermatologists. My grandmother made a version of her scented lotion by using lemons.

INGREDIENTS

> 2 cups of lotion
>
> 2 ounces of your favorite
>   fragrance

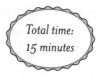

*Total time:
15 minutes*

Pour the lotion into a bowl (make sure to keep the original container for later). Now add the scent. You can either follow the Orange Glow recipe or go to a health food store and buy some essential fragrance oils. My favorite scents are orange, lemon, mango, and vanilla. Mix your scent and lotion base.

Once your body lotion is well blended, you're ready to bottle your creation. Either pour it back into the original container or reuse some old ones. Be sure your empty bottles are clean before using them to store your new creations. Using a small kitchen funnel, slowly pour the lotion from the bowl to the bottle.

Chapter Five

Countdown to the Big Event

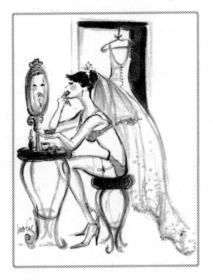

One reason clients come to see me is to "beautify" themselves for an upcoming event. Maybe a high school reunion is coming up in a few days. Indulge me while I paint a picture. You feel a bit bloated and your skin isn't in the best shape. Whether it's a reunion (with Facebook, do we even need high school reunions anymore?) or a big birthday, or maybe you're meeting your boyfriend's parents for the first time—whatever the scenario, you want to look your best. Well, don't panic. Ukrainian help is on the way!

My babushka was as cool as a cucumber under

pressure. She would say just be yourself. When you relax, everything else falls into place.

This chapter is designed to get you ready for the big event from head to toe. Most of the recipes are formulated to plump up the face with special ingredients for this very special occasion. In Hollywood, clients are supposed to look good for that big night — so they rely heavily on these recipes. Everyone wants to make a good impression when they walk in that room or down the red carpet. These recipes are designed to wow the crowd!

A plastic surgeon friend recently explained to me how his practice has been changing in the last few years. In the past he was performing more surgeries, but now his business is shifting toward using fillers such as Restalyne and Juvéderm to put volume back in the face. When I look at the famous actresses of the fifties, many of them were indeed beauties, but as they got older, plastic surgeons would pull their faces too tight. We still see women with bad surgery, but today volumizing is the trend rather than cutting and pulling.

My clients often refer to my masks as natural fillers. They leave women looking younger, healthier, and more relaxed (but not overly relaxed in that airbrushed, Hollywood sort of way). Think of these recipes as natural Restalyne, or collagen without the painful injections.

My clients rely on me to make them look good before any big event. They report back about the endless compliments they get about their skin while walking down the red carpet at the Oscars or at a movie premiere. It makes me incredibly proud to think these recipes work so well on some of the greatest beauties in the world—women who are extremely selective about what they'll put on their skin.

This chapter offers perfect recipes to use before heading out on a big date, going back to the high school reunion, or attending a wedding (maybe it's your own). One of my clients did three of these recipes in one day. It may sound a little excessive, but she looked great. No need to do so many, though, since one will definitely do the trick.

Sunken Soufflé

Watermelon and honeydew are ideal ways to naturally reduce water weight. We all want to jump into a dress looking our best, but some days there's a little extra something here or there, even if you didn't eat that much the day before! This next recipe will set you up for that little black dress.

INGREDIENTS

1 slice watermelon

1 slice honeydew

Total time:
5 minutes

Place these two fruits into a blender and put it on high for 2 minutes. Drink it up. Enjoy!

Babushka's Beauty Tip:

Eating cucumbers also helps prevent
water retention. Cucumbers are very
effective for swelling under the eyes and
for sunburn as well.

Date Soufflé

Whenever anyone went out on a date, my mother would suggest this soufflé since it tightens the skin and gives it a gorgeous glow. Even if you don't have a date, you just may attract one with this recipe.

STEP ONE

INGREDIENTS

Total time:
20 minutes

½ teaspoon baking soda

½ teaspoon sugar

½ teaspoon shaving cream

Mix the ingredients together in a small bowl and massage in the skin for 5 minutes. Rinse with cool tap water and then rinse again with mineral water. You won't believe how it can remove dead skin from the surface, which prepares your skin for the next step.

STEP TWO

1 egg (Use the egg white for oily skin or the
    yolk for dry skin.)

1 tablespoon sour cream

2 drops vitamin E

In a small bowl, stir the ingredients together. Apply to the face and leave on for 10–15 minutes. Rinse with lukewarm tap water.

The Close-Up Soufflé

My clients insist on this recipe before a big photo shoot. As a child, I had no idea about the size of one's pores, but my babushka was obsessed with having small ones. This was one of my grandmother's favorite recipes because she felt it could really change the texture of the skin. As we get older, our pores get larger. This soufflé is the perfect way to combat this problem. If you're going to have your picture taken for the big event, start shrinking those pores a week before the big night. You can do this twice in one week.

Total time:
15 minutes

INGREDIENTS

1 egg white

1 tablespoon lemon juice

2 tablespoons oatmeal

1 shredded tomato

Place all the ingredients in a blender and puree until it has a thick sour cream–like texture (the oatmeal will leave it a little lumpy). Apply the mixture to the skin and leave it on for 10 minutes. Rinse off the soufflé with warm tap water.

> ### Babushka's Beauty Tip:
>
> Hollywood actresses love combining the Date
> Soufflé and the Close-Up Soufflé. Do the
> Close-Up Soufflé first. Follow it up with the
> Date Soufflé. Your skin will look flawless!

Romance Soufflé

I love chocolate. It's one of my biggest weaknesses. Put potato chips in front of me I could care less, but give me dark chocolate—covered raisins and forget about it! Chocolate has several ingredients that can potentially sweeten the skin. Also remember that cocoa is a good antioxidant.

This next recipe is so yummy, you may be tempted to eat it, but put it on your face first! Try this mask when you want to look perfect for that certain someone.

Total time: 25 minutes

INGREDIENTS

⅓ cup dark cocoa

3 tablespoons heavy cream

¼ cup honey

2 tablespoons oatmeal

2 tablespoons milk (for later)

Run the oatmeal through a food processor or blender until it becomes a powder. Mix all the ingredients together (with the exception of the milk). Apply to your face and leave on for 20 minutes. Rinse it off with lukewarm water. Then rinse your skin with milk. Use a cotton ball to apply it, and follow up with water.

✳ Aspirin ✳

*A*ll this talk about the big event may be giving you a headache. But aspirin isn't just for pain relief. While it's a drug used to relieve minor aches, pains, fever, and inflammation, aspirin can actually have a number of other uses as well. But if you're allergic to aspirin, don't use this on your skin, hair, or clothing either.

Did you know aspirin can...

1. **Remove perspiration stains.** Simply crush 2 aspirins and mix the powder with half a cup of warm water. Soak the stain in the solution for 2–3 hours to reveal a cleaner garment.

2. **Treat calluses on your feet.** Soften your feet by grinding 6 aspirins into a powder and adding half a teaspoon of lemon juice and water. Apply the paste around your feet and wrap them in a warm towel or plastic bag.

3. **Control dandruff.** Try crushing 2 tablets and add them to your normal amount of shampoo each time you wash your hair. Leave the mixture on for 2 minutes, then rinse with water.

4. **Reduce inflammation from an insect bite.** Simply wet your skin and rub an aspirin over the spot to control the inflammation.

5. **Relieve the pain of a toothache.** Put a tablet of baby aspirin on the affected tooth and let it dissolve.

6. **Stop the bleeding from shaving.** When you cut yourself shaving, it's always tough to stop the

(cont.)

✳ ASPIRIN (CONT.) ✳

bleeding, but if you dissolve an aspirin in some warm water and then apply the mixture on a cotton ball, the bleeding will stop quickly.

7. **Help cut flowers last longer.** This is a great trick to keep roses and other cut flowers fresh longer. Put a crushed aspirin in the water before adding your flowers.

Wedding Soufflé

Whether you're the bride, the bridesmaid, the mother of the bride, or simply a guest, this is a brilliant mask for a wedding. (Remember, single women, weddings are a great place to meet men.) One way to get that beautiful, youthful glow in your skin is to get the blood flowing.

INGREDIENTS

Total time: 10 minutes

    1 teaspoon olive oil

    1 teaspoon mustard

    ½ teaspoon tomato juice

    ½ teaspoon vinegar

    1 tablespoon (unbleached) white flour

    ⅛ cup buttermilk (for later)

Mix all the ingredients except the buttermilk in a small bowl. Stir and apply the mask to the skin by rubbing it in your hands like a lotion and then spreading it on the face. Leave it on for 5–10 minutes. (Don't worry if you feel a little tingle on your face: It's designed to get the blood flowing. But never leave anything on if it begins feeling uncomfortable.) Rinse with lukewarm water and pat skin dry. Follow with the buttermilk by simply soaking a cotton ball in it and applying it all over the skin. Rinse off after a few minutes.

Wedding Anniversary Soufflé

This is also a good one for the big event since your skin will be glowing! I love this soufflé because it gives immediate results. If you have sensitive skin, don't use as much pumpkin. This can be a little strong and you'll definitely feel it on the skin, which is why I've added a teaspoon of honey. This recipe is a bit more complicated than the others but well worth it. I suggest cleaning out a pumpkin and boiling it up. However, I do have clients who cheat and use canned pumpkin. Whichever you choose, the pumpkin must be cooked.

INGREDIENTS

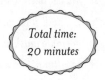

Total time:
20 minutes

¼ cup fresh papaya, mashed

½ cup pumpkin

I egg

I teaspoon honey

2 tablespoons milk (for later)

Cut the papaya in half and scoop out the fruit minus the seeds. Now throw the pumpkin, papaya, egg, and honey into the blender. Mix it all on high for I minute, apply on your face, and leave it on for IO minutes. Rinse with water. Now grab a cotton ball, dip it in the milk, and apply to your face. Leave it on for a few minutes before rinsing with warm water. Since you'll have extra, add a quarter teaspoon of vodka and store the leftover mix in the refrigerator.

Stress Soufflé

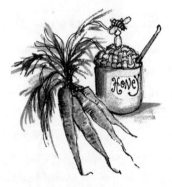

If you've been traveling before your big night, then definitely try this. It will put much-needed moisture back in your face. This honey antiwrinkle mask will plump up the volume and reduce wrinkles. Honey is the ultimate moisturizer and loaded with vitamin A. My babushka was such a fan of honey. She used it in everything. Carrots are also a good source of vitamin C and a powerful antioxidant that help fight premature aging. It also aids in producing collagen, which helps the skin look young and taut.

INGREDIENTS

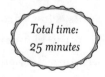

Total time: 25 minutes

    1 tablespoon honey

    ½ teaspoon fresh carrot juice

    ¼ teaspoon baking soda

Combine the honey, carrot juice, and baking soda in a small bowl and stir well. Apply the mask all over the face. Leave it on for 20 minutes. Remove the mask with lukewarm water. Dip a cotton ball in the mineral water, and apply it all over the face and neck.

Baby Shower Soufflé

My mother loved making any kind of strawberry or blueberry recipes. Rather than craving chocolate when she was pregnant with us, she craved berries. Strawberries basically act as an alpha hydroxy acid — a brilliant substance for getting rid of dead skin cells to make room for new youthful skin.

This recipe can perk up the most battered, weathered skin. I remember my grandmother used it on one of her friends, whose skin was dull, and we watched the glow suddenly come back.

This is also a favorite for my model/actress clients who need to look refreshed after a late night. So if you happen to be out late the night before your big event, definitely use this recipe.

INGREDIENTS

½ teaspoon talc-free baby powder

4 medium-size strawberries

2 tablespoons mineral water (for later)

Total time: 7 minutes

This recipe is as simple as they come! Put the ingredients (powder and strawberries) into a blender on high for 2 minutes. (It will have the texture of a smoothie, but don't drink it!) Apply to the skin for 5 minutes. Rinse off with mineral water.

Graduation Soufflé

Can you believe they're already graduating? Or maybe it's your gradu-ation. Look your best. This will leave your skin feeling rejuvenated! The enzymes in papaya are amazing for the skin. And buttermilk is another wonderful ingredient. Mix the two together and you have a mask that will transform your skin! I have a few actresses who say this simple recipe gives them the most amazing glow and leaves the skin feeling like butter . . . or should I say . . . buttermilk!

INGREDIENTS

   2 tablespoons papaya

   1 tablespoon buttermilk

Total time:
About
25 minutes

Mix the ingredients and throw them in the blender for 1 minute on high. Next, apply the mask on your face for 15–20 minutes. Wash it off with lukewarm water. Pat your skin dry.

Reunion Soufflé

Want to look younger at the reunion? Check this recipe out! Papaya is the best natural face-lift money can buy. Look on the back of many big cosmetic brands and you'll notice that they use papaya in everything from peels to lotions. It is full of enzymes, minerals, and vitamins. And pineapple is a brilliant way to exfoliate the skin. This recipe will give the face a natural lift and a gorgeous glow! Don't be surprised if someone asks, "What have you done?"

INGREDIENTS

½ cup fresh pineapple

½ papaya (cut up in cubes)

I tablespoon honey

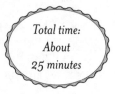

Total time:
About
25 minutes

Put the fruit in the blender on high for I minute, add the honey, and puree another 30 seconds. Place on the face and neck for 20 minutes. Rinse off with lukewarm water.

✳ FACE-OFF FOR THE BIG EVENT ✳

Here are a number of things you should always avoid — but especially the week before the big event. It will make a real difference in your appearance.

1. **Turn down the heat.** I love hot showers! There is nothing better. Back in the Ukraine hot showers were considered a major luxury, but in reality hot water is bad for the skin because it's so drying.

2. **Be caffeine-free.** This can be difficult, but it's important to watch your intake. My clients want their morning coffee. I do, too. One cup of coffee isn't going to bring out wrinkles instantly, but if you drink it all day, it can deprive your body and skin of water and certain nutrients, which promotes the formation of wrinkles.

3. **Don't dry out.** If you live in a desert like Arizona or Palm Springs, where there's little humidity, you should definitely invest in a vaporizer or humidifier.

(cont.)

✳ FACE-OFF FOR THE BIG EVENT (CONT.) ✳

Even if you live in a more humid climate but leave the heat on all winter, pull out the humidifier.

4. **Stay sugarless.** This is another tough rule to follow. I love chocolate, especially dark chocolate. However, recent studies point to evidence that too much sugar can accelerate the aging process. I'm not saying stay away completely. Again, moderation is the key.

5. **Drop the soap.** Have you ever washed your face and felt as though it was going to fall off afterward because it was so dry? Cleansers and soaps don't have to be drying to work.

Chapter Six

Open Your Eyes

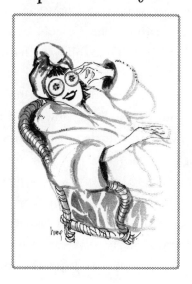

"You look tired." Those are three words I despise hearing. I often feel like replying, "You *are* tired!" Even if someone does look tired, no one should ever utter those rude words. Unfortunately, when those words are directed your way, it's usually because your eyes appear puffy or tired. Maybe it's a lack of sleep? Quite possibly allergies are causing those dark circles? Or maybe too much salt the night before? Whatever the reason, it can be quite a difficult situation to cover up. My babushka always believed the eyes never lied. Nor did the undereyes.

There are many different remedies for treating puffy

eyes in the morning. My babushka had three weapons against puffy eyes and dark circles. Some of them you've heard before, but there's an extra trick on this list: Put two metal teaspoons in the fridge before you go to bed and place them on your eyes (for 10 minutes if they're puffy) in the morning. The icy cool of the metal will relieve sore, tired eyes. Then follow with one of these:

* **Frozen peas.** Put frozen peas in a ziplock bag and lay it across your eyes to bring down puffiness. I have a number of clients who do this trick first thing in the morning.
* **Green tea bags.** Dip two tea bags in cold water and apply on each eye. It will bring down puffiness and the caffeine will shrink blood vessels.
* **Cucumbers.** Cut two ½-inch thick slices of a refrigerated cucumber and apply one on each eye for 5 minutes to reduce puffiness.

Crow's-feet, dark circles, and bags! Those are the three areas most women complain about when it comes to the eyes. I have some surefire recipes to help in these areas and more. My clients are often amazed at how well these recipes work. I will put them up to store-bought products any day. The benefits from items such as potatoes, cucumbers, cabbage, and bananas will change the way you view everyday fruits and veggies. Trust me, the recipes in this chapter will open your eyes to a whole new world of beauty!

~ DARK CIRCLES AND BAGS ~

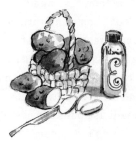

Potato Poof

Potatoes were my grandmother's thing. She loved to eat them and use them to remove dark circles and puffiness. The skin around and under the eyes is the thinnest and most sensitive on the entire body. Puffiness under (or above) the eyes is quite common. Sliced potatoes work wonders for puffiness and dark circles. To banish bags, simply put on a potato and poof . . . the puffiness is gone.

INGREDIENTS

1 potato

1 tablespoon vitamin E

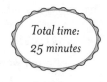

Total time: 25 minutes

Here is the brilliant part of this recipe—there is no cooking involved (but don't get too used to it!). Wash the potato well. Cut two ⅛-inch slices from the middle (save the rest for the next several nights.) Apply one on top of each eye for 20 minutes. Remove the potatoes and apply vitamin E in a circular motion around and under the eyes.

Babushka's Beauty Tip:

Many of us have heard how Preparation H works so well on bags and dark circles. Back in the day some enterprising young models used Preparation H after a hard night of partying to get rid of dark circles. But believe me and my clients — potatoes are safer and more effective! I have a model client who will use potatoes over Preparation H any day.

Banish Bags

Vitamin K can kick out dark circles! Known as the best vitamin for removing dark circles, vitamin K heals damaged capillaries and minimizes the pooling of blood under the eyes, a major factor in causing dark circles. The thinner the skin near the eye, the more visible the dark circles will appear if this isn't done. Dark circles won't disappear overnight with vitamin K. But with patience, you'll see a big difference. These ingredients all contain the big K.

INGREDIENTS

2 cups water

1 bunch basil

1 bunch parsley leaves

3 pieces of lettuce

3 pieces of cabbage

Total time: 28 minutes

Boil the water in a pan and throw in the remaining ingredients. Simmer for 18 minutes and then strain the liquid and pour it into a reusable container. Apply with a washcloth or cotton ball under the eyes and leave on for 10 minutes. Repeat daily. This mixture must be refrigerated. Add a ½ teaspoon of vodka or wine to make this dark circle buster last a month!

Lighten Up!

These next three recipes are fantastic for diminishing dark circles. They all contain ingredients that are most likely in your home. I would alternate these recipes every couple of days. In a few weeks, you'll notice those dark circles are lightening up!

INGREDIENTS

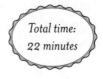

Total time: 22 minutes

    1 tablespoon white flour

    1 tablespoon milk

    ½ teaspoon hydrogen peroxide

Throw all the ingredients into a tiny bowl and stir with a spoon. Apply the mixture under your eyes for 20 minutes and then rinse with a little buttermilk. If you don't have buttermilk, simply rinse with water.

Light Cream

INGREDIENTS

Total time: 22 minutes

    1 teaspoon sour cream

    1 teaspoon honey

    ½ teaspoon lemon

Mix all the ingredients in a small bowl and apply under the eyes for 20 minutes. Rinse with warm water and pat dry.

Put on Peroxide

INGREDIENTS

1 teaspoon mayo

10 drops hydrogen peroxide

10 drops lemon

Total time: 22 minutes

Mix the ingredients in a small bowl and apply under the eyes for 20 minutes. Not only will this recipe lighten the skin, but it will increase the blood to the area and diminish fine lines.

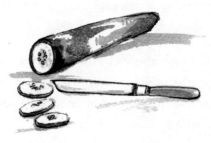

Cucumber Circles

Cucumbers are a brilliant way to remove dark circles! In old movies we often see women on the couch with cucumbers over their eyes. They did it back then because it worked. The cucumbers will help lighten up dark circles and puffiness under the eyes.

INGREDIENTS

1 cucumber

2 tablespoons almond oil

Total time:
30 minutes

Soak two slices (about ¼-inch thick) of cucumbers in the almond oil for 15 minutes. Pat the cucumbers dry. Once you've done that, simply place them over your eyes (while lying down). Keep them over your eyes for about 10 minutes.

Babushka's Beauty Tip:

Bananas are a great way to lighten up the undereyes. Simply smash one up and apply for 20 minutes. The potassium will diminish wrinkles and dark circles.

CROW'S-FEET

I was at Whole Foods the other day with a forty-something-year-old girlfriend combing the skin care aisle. My friend turned to me and asked, "What's that young girl doing buying antiaging eye cream?" I turned to my friend and said, "She's investing in her future by snapping up a little wrinkle insurance early." Good for her!

Nothing is worse than watching those lines come in on the sides of our eyes. You know the lines—those dreaded crow's-feet! Unfortunately crow's-feet are the first wrinkles to appear on a woman's face. Funny enough, my babushka believed eyes shouldn't show a woman's age. But let's face it—this is a tricky area since it's quite susceptible to fine lines and wrinkles. Here are a few tips:

1. Avoid using heavy amounts of foundation or powder around crow's-feet. It's better to use a little foundation only where you need it. I always wear makeup under my eyes to cover dark circles, but that's about it.

2. Avoid too much sun. Need I say more?

3. Avoid smoking. It's so aging!

4. Wear sunglasses—big ones!

5. Remove your eye makeup every night.

Heard It Through the Grapevine

Since ancient times, grapes have been used for cosmetic reasons. Many old recipes call for grape juice to reduce wrinkles. (Yes, through the years, people have been obsessed with erasing those fine lines.) Grapes contain something called malic acid, which is an important alpha hydroxy acid in many beauty products.

INGREDIENT

   20 green Thompson seedless
   grapes

Total time:
25 minutes

This is a perfect home remedy for wrinkles. Put the grapes in a mixer, put on high for a minute, and pour the juice out. Apply this juice to your face using a cotton ball and let it stay on for 20 minutes. Rinse with warm water to get the best results.

Babushka's Beauty Tip:

One actress has me make up this potion every few weeks. After applying it in the morning, she does another little grape trick as well. Simply cut a grape in half and rub it softly around the crow's-feet—it's brilliant for diminishing wrinkles!

Oy, the Soy!

Chinese women believe soy is very good to fight aging. This next recipe does wonders for reducing fine lines and crow's-feet. I have a client who demands this treatment after a sleepless night or a long weekend. She swears it takes ten years off her face. I agree!

INGREDIENTS

¼ cup soybeans, soaked
overnight in 1 cup of water

1 tablespoon whole milk

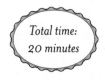

Total time:
20 minutes

In the morning blend the soybeans into a paste in the blender. Then throw in the milk and blend for another minute. Place under the eyes for 15 minutes. It is brilliant at diminishing crow's-feet and fine lines.

Almond Joy

One of the most common complaints I hear is, "Why do my crow's-feet seem so prominent on certain days?" Well, there are a number of explanations. Maybe you were traveling and the skin is a bit dehydrated. You lost a little weight, which can sometimes be a bit aging. Or you simply didn't get enough sleep the night before. This next recipe may just put that complaining to rest.

INGREDIENTS

    2 tablespoons grated cocoa butter

    2 tablespoons coconut oil

    1 tablespoon almond oil

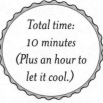

Total time: 10 minutes (Plus an hour to let it cool.)

Combine the ingredients and place the mixture in the microwave for 20 seconds or less. (Be sure to watch it.) The cocoa butter needs to fully melt, but you don't want it to start to bubble. Mix it up, pour it into a tiny container, and let it sit for an hour so it can cool. Apply it under the eyes before bed. Stick the extra mix in the refrigerator.

LOVELY LASHES

Raya's Revitalash

Do you remember when Revitalash was all the rage? It's a particularly strong chemical women put on their eyelashes to make them grow. I frequently use castor oil and find it basically does the same thing. My grandmother always said, "This makes lashes grow like that of a cow." A

*nightly brushing with castor oil is an old-fashioned treatment to pro-
duce long, luscious lashes.*

INGREDIENT

1 teaspoon castor oil

Total time:
2 minutes

Before bed, dip a cotton swab in the castor oil. Now place
the oil-soaked swab on the upper and lower lash line
and then all over the lashes. Go to sleep and be patient
with the results . . . I promise in a few months your lashes
will look incredible! One of my clients' motto was unless
she goes under or gets something in prescription form, it
doesn't really work, but she believes (with patience) castor
oil is amazing.

Remove That Mascara!

Besides sun, do you want to know the worst thing for
crow's-feet? Sleeping with your makeup on all night! Who
hasn't woken up to a full face of makeup? This isn't a good
habit. Sure those mascara smudges can look sexy in the
morning, but leaving a thick coat of mascara on overnight
isn't good for the eyes or the skin. (Call me neurotic, but
leaving mascara on overnight is also a bacterial disaster.)
Not to mention it can spotlight any fine lines or creases
(like women need any more grief!). Lashes will also
become brittle and break off, which will leave a gap on
your lash line. Not exactly attractive! I have a great, easy
recipe for removing mascara. It's something you'll want
to use every night.

Take It All Off

Even if you have a makeup remover you love, please try this! It's simple, easy, and does the trick like nothing else I've ever used before.

INGREDIENTS

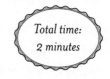

Total time:
2 minutes

1 tablespoon olive oil
(extra virgin)
2 tablespoons canola oil

Combine the oils in a small bowl. Dip a cotton ball or swab into the mixture. Gently wipe your lash line and move it forward. Do this a couple of times. Then go back and clean up the smudges on the lid and under the eye. Rinse your face with warm water, throw on your cleanser, and continue your nightly routine. There are eye makeup removers selling for over $50! Why, when it's in the kitchen? Put the extra liquid in a reusable container and use it for the next couple of weeks. When removing mascara, always remember: Don't rub too hard around the eyes. Using oil will help the mascara slip off easier and doesn't pull on the lashes.

Chapter Seven

Lip Service

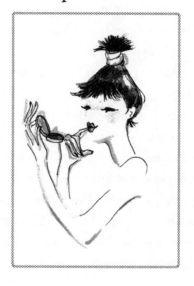

$\mathcal{M}$y grandmother was famous for saying, "Lips are the most important part of the face. They are used for everything from speech to food." She loved talking and eating—they were her two favorite things!

Lips are the ultimate symbol of not just sensuality, but sexuality. My babushka believed lips were the ultimate way to communicate with a man—from producing a flirty pout to puckering up!

Just look at the millions of dollars spent each year on lipsticks, glosses, enhancers, and other products designed to give the illusion of an Angelina pout. Without knowing it, when we think of beautiful, youthful smiles, we picture full, soft, smooth, wrinkle-free lips.

Attaining the defined, sexy, and sensuous look is often a matter of genetics. And even if you're lucky enough to be blessed with the perfect pout, the aging process can take its toll. Unfortunately it causes lips to recede and thin over time, which explains why women spend millions each year on products such as collagen and Juvéderm to enhance the lips.

That's because the lips are actually one of the first places on your face to reveal age. Like the eyes, lips' outer layer gets thinner as we lose collagen with age. With time, lips become dry and are more susceptible to wrinkling. My grandmother was obsessed with keeping her lips moist. She couldn't stand to see the lines above her lips. My babushka wasn't really into physical exercise, but she did sort of exercise her lips each morning by doing three simple moves:

* **The minute massage.** It's really quite simple: Just place your thumb on the inside of your upper lip and then take your forefinger and place it on the outside of your upper lip and massage the entire area for 1 minute. This will give the lips a little volume before adding your lipstick. Some days I put a dab of mayonnaise on each finger to add moisture. When our lips are dry, they appear smaller.

* **Brush your teeth; brush your lips.** First thing in the morning when you wake up and brush your

teeth, don't leave out your lips. It may sound crazy but it gets the blood moving to the area and it will pump your lips up.

✳ **Black tea stick.** Saturate a black tea bag with warm water. Press over clean lips for 5 minutes. Black tea is high in tannic acid, which retains moisture and keeps lips smooth and taut. You'll perk them up!

My grandmother knew that when the lips are dry, they look smaller. Although she loved her native home, she despised the cold weather and was highly aware of how those brutal winters could be aging. But she had many tricks for the skin. We were under strict orders to always keep petroleum jelly on our lips at all times. Baby oil was another good trick to moisten the lips before braving the bitter cold. They both worked. Most kids my age had dry, cracked lips, whereas mine were always soft and smooth, thanks to my babushka.

LIP MOISTURIZERS

Honey Lips

This next recipe will infuse the lips with moisture and vitamins. When you mix honey, avocado, mango, and toothpaste, it's a brilliant combination! Just try it — it will make the lips look young and smooth.

INGREDIENTS

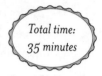

Total time:
35 minutes

1 tablespoon shredded mango

1 tablespoon smashed avocado

1 tablespoon honey

¾ tablespoon of any toothpaste

1 small surgical pad (If you don't have one, then use
a paper towel you've cut into a 2 × 2-inch pad.)

Mash up the mango and avocado until they become a creamy mixture. Now throw in the honey and toothpaste and mix everything together well in a blender for 1 minute. Soak the surgical pad (lip patch) in the mixture for 10 minutes. Leave the pad on your lips for 20 minutes. It's the ultimate moisturizer.

Apple Infusion

I eat three apples on any given day. They are so delicious — while satisfying my sweet tooth, they are also high in fiber. Apples are also incredibly moisturizing for the lips. This simple treatment will light up your lips. It's a good mask to use before bed. You'll love how your lips look in the morning. It will supply vitamin C and moisture, and putting on lipstick will never seem so easy.

INGREDIENTS

Total time:
10 minutes

1 slice green apple (about ½ inch
in width)

1 teaspoon butter

After you put on your cleanser and moisturizer, throw on this mask. Massage the lips with a slice of an apple for 5 minutes, then apply butter on top. Don't wash anything off. Leave it on overnight. When you wake up in the morning, you'll want to lick your lips since they'll taste so good!

Forget Flaky Lips

My grandmother used this recipe on so many women during those brutal winters in the Ukraine. This next recipe is brilliant to use before bed and as soon as you wake up in the morning. These are four common ingredients in every household and they will smooth out lips better than any balm. In addition to moisturizing, the sugar in the recipe will help exfoliate and get rid of any of those unwanted flakes on your lips. Suddenly your lips will be ready for a little color.

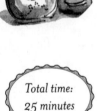

INGREDIENTS

    1 teaspoon olive oil

    1 teaspoon honey

    2 teaspoons sugar

    ½ teaspoon lemon juice

Total time: 25 minutes

Mix the ingredients in a small bowl and apply on the lips. Keep the mixture on for 20 minutes and then wash off. Now put some gloss on those smooth lips!

Babushka's Beauty Tip:

Scrub away dry skin by mixing Epsom salt with petroleum jelly. This treatment will also give your lips a bit of plumping since salt retains water.

Pineapple C

Pineapple is high in the enzyme bromelain and it's an antioxidant—both of which help it play a major role in the body's healing process. This recipe will soften the lips and give them a little boost since it contains tons of vitamin C, which helps the body boost the production of collagen.

INGREDIENT

1 slice pineapple

Total time: 1 minute

Before bed rub the pineapple all over the lips. Don't rinse it off; instead apply petroleum jelly on top of it and go to sleep with that sweet smell on your lips.

Oil and E

Talk about pouring moisture back into your lips. You'll love this concoction. Put it on before bed and you won't believe the change in your lips. They'll be moist and ready for some lipstick. I find vitamin E protects my lips for hours. I always use it during the winter months to ensure my lips stay soft and smooth.

INGREDIENTS

   1 tablespoon honey

   1 teaspoon of olive oil

   ½ teaspoon vitamin E

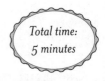

Total time:
5 minutes

In a small bowl combine the honey, olive oil, and vitamin E.
Mix them all together and store in an old lip gloss container
or keep covered in a small bowl. Apply every night and you
won't believe the difference. Expiration date: one month.

Coconut Gloss

*Aloe vera gel and coconut oil are my favorites for the lips. This recipe
has both. You'll love it! There are so many people who complain about
the addictive nature of lip balms. There are no harmful preservatives in
this gloss and you'll adore the way it moisturizes the lips!*

INGREDIENTS

   1 teaspoon aloe vera gel

   ½ teaspoon coconut oil

   1 teaspoon petroleum jelly

Total time:
2 minutes
(Add an hour to let
it freeze.)

Mix together in a glass bowl and store in either a small
Tupperware or an old lip balm container. Put the mix-
ture in the freezer for an hour and then it's ready to use!
Store it in the freezer to make it last longer.

Sweetening the Pot

*This may be one of the easiest and most satisfying of all the recipes. You
are basically making a gloss out of three simple ingredients, and there's*

*a bonus — it tastes amazing on your lips! It also offers up a little color.
It's really quite pretty.*

INGREDIENTS

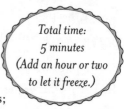

Total time:
5 minutes
(Add an hour or two
to let it freeze.)

1 teaspoon Aquaphor
(a healing ointment
available at most drugstores;
petroleum jelly can be used
as a substitute)

2 dark chocolate chips

1 drop peppermint oil

Melt the chocolate chips in a glass dish and mix with
Aquaphor and peppermint oil. Put inside an old lip ointment container. Now drop in the freezer (the gloss will be
ready in 1–2 hours). Vanilla and spearmint oil are brilliant sweeteners, as well.

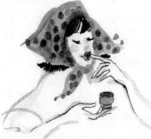

MIX YOUR COLOR

Turn a boring balm into a creative color. Why, you ask?
Quite simply because it's fun and easy. Add a drop of honey
to each of these and you won't believe the final product.

1. **Beet juice.** Add a few drops of beet juice into a plain lip balm and you're sitting pretty with tinted gloss.

2. **Carrot juice.** Add a few drops of carrot juice to a lip balm and suddenly you'll produce color and moisturize the lips.

3. **Red grapes.** These will apply a little color as well.

Carrot Kisses

Here's another brilliant way to add a little color to the lips (I think this is best on blondes). Since carrots tend to stain the lips, you won't believe the results. In addition to lip stain, the honey will act as a moisturizer. It will diminish wrinkles above the lip line as well.

INGREDIENTS

2–3 large carrots

4½ tablespoons honey

Total time:
25 minutes

Cook the carrots (boil or steam until they're soft), then put them in the blender to make a perfect puree. Mix with honey. Apply gently to the skin, and wait 10 minutes. Rinse off with cool water.

Lipstick

Do you realize that the average women ingests up to 4 pounds of lipstick or gloss in a lifetime? Just think of the lipstick you observe on your glass after having a drink or a cup of coffee. Unfortunately it's entering your body, too. I'm not trying to scare you but to prove how obsessed we are with our lips. Truthfully, it hasn't stopped me from wearing lipstick at night.

My over-forty clients often complain about wrinkles around their lips. To add insult to injury, applying lipstick can accentuate the wrinkles. Since darker colors often highlight the wrinkles around the lips, it's best to stick to nudes rather than reds. Who knew lipstick was so complicated?

I love lipstick but despise some of the common problems that go along with the application. If that's the case for you, then you'll love these next tips from a top Hollywood makeup artist. Forget about throwing away broken lipstick or putting up with it coming off too quickly. These are some simple solutions to such common lipstick problems.

 1. **To make your lipstick stay on longer,** simply put foundation on your lips and follow up with a little powder. Now apply the lipstick and a little more powder on top of it and then go over it again with lipstick. You're golden for a couple of hours!

 2. **Broken lipstick happens to the best of us.** Your lipstick suddenly breaks and now you wonder what to do with it. Is the lipstick going in the trash? Not so fast! Get a pill container (you know the one with the seven days of the week) and simply break off a part of the stick and smash it inside. It's kind of brilliant since it gives you an opportunity

to put in other colors as well (even those that aren't broken). Seven colors to be exact. You can apply with your finger or a brush. Another advantage of lipstick palettes is they can easily plop right inside your handbag. Now you can choose from several different colors rather than bringing along just one shade. It also allows for mixing colors together and creating something new. This is an old trick professional makeup artists use to transport lipstick.

3. Add a little shine to make lips appear bigger. After applying lipstick, put a dab of a lighter gloss in the middle of the lip to put out a little pout.

4. Before applying lipstick, use a little cream. Many top models prepare their mouth by dipping a cotton swab in a rich moisturizer and rubbing it across their lips to loosen dry flakes. Pat with a tissue and apply lipstick.

Chapter Eight

Well-Tressed

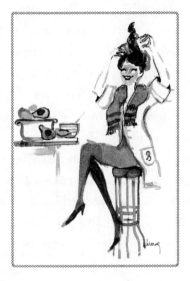

On my last trip to Moscow, I was walking down the street and couldn't help noticing all the glamazons strutting along. This was a different Moscow than the one I'd left over a decade ago. Leggy Russian women in high heels giggled as they tossed their long thick hair from side to side. Even though the temperature in January didn't reflect it, Russia was hot!

Although life has dramatically changed, the love affair Russian women have with long locks is very much the same. My grandmother was a fan of long hair and couldn't understand why any woman would ever have short hair (personally I love both). From the time I can remember, my babushka wore her salt and pepper hair in a long braid down her back.

She had beautiful, healthy hair but didn't believe in rinsing money down the drain. But we all do it every day—spending billions of dollars a year on hair care products. And the obsession with hair isn't restricted to women.

A friend of mine was telling me how he watched a story on the news about men who were seeking a rather unusual animal treatment in an effort to stimulate their failing follicles. After trekking to an obscure location, patients lined up to pay for the privilege of having a donkey lick the top of their heads—all in the hopes of sprouting new hair. (Talk about putting a price on your head!) Upon hearing this, I began researching the subject and found cows will perform the same service. Who knew?

A few days later, a client of mine came in to do a little waxing and suddenly blurted out, "Does my upper lip seem more hairy this time?" "No," I replied. "Why are you asking?" In an agitated tone she began explaining how a bad haircut left her desperately seeking a treatment of seaweed and kelp (directly from the ocean) in hopes of growing her luxurious locks back quickly. It didn't work and she was paranoid it might have sprouted more facial hair.

This isn't something happening just in the United States. Hair is an international affair. All around the world, people are willing to try just about any obscure treatment to hang on to it:

* In Russia there is a well-known recipe of vodka, honey, and onion. Men and women put it all over their heads!
* In China they use a kidney tonic and acupuncture to stimulate hair growth.
* In Europe they prefer nettle root extract.
* The ever-efficient Japanese have a different method in which patients listen to their favorite music wearing special headphones that produce a low-frequency current said to stimulate the scalp and get blood flowing to hair follicles.

Some of these "treatments" sound a bit dubious to say the least (although my babushka believed onion skin is remarkable for hair growth). But it proves that people will go to great lengths for their hair.

So let's get primping. You will love your new locks!

I'll Take Mayo and Mustard!

These next two recipes are fantastic if you're trying to grow out your hair. I work with an actress who loved her cute, sassy haircut until her new boyfriend begged her to grow it long. Rather than put in extensions, she decided to wait it out. She is convinced this next recipe expedited the process.

INGREDIENTS

- I tablespoon mayo
- I tablespoon mustard
- I dash cayenne pepper

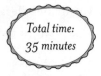

Total time: 35 minutes

Put everything together in a small bowl and stir it up. Rub the mixture through your hands and then all over your scalp. After 30 minutes, shampoo, dry, and go! Do this recipe once a week and alternate a couple days later with the next recipe.

C-Squared

INGREDIENTS

- 2 tablespoons castor oil
- 2 tablespoons cognac

Total time: 30 minutes

Mix up the ingredients in a small bowl and apply all over your scalp. Wash out with shampoo after 25 minutes.

Hair Sprout

There's nothing worse than a bad haircut! Rather than glue in hair extensions, why not give it a little patience? It won't happen overnight but it will help those locks grow a little faster.

INGREDIENTS

- 2 tablespoons aloe vera
- 2 tablespoons honey

Total time: 25 minutes

Mix and apply all over the scalp and let it sit for 20 minutes. Rinse with warm water and shampoo out.

> ### Babushka's Beauty Tip:
>
> My grandmother always believed putting olive oil in the hair for 30 minutes twice a week was a brilliant way to promote hair growth. Also the less you wash your hair, the better. Allowing the natural oils to get into the scalp is good for the process. I have a client who swears prenatal vitamins are also brilliant for making the hair grow.

Volumize

My clients often complain about thin hair and put in extensions to add volume. One of my clients didn't have the heart to tell a friend her hair was thinning. She asked if I'd suggest she get extensions. Instead I suggested this next recipe. It gives the hair a little boost!

INGREDIENTS

Total time:
45 minutes

1 egg yolk

1 teaspoon of apple cider

Mix the two ingredients together in a small bowl. Add the contents all over the scalp and keep on your hair for 40 minutes if possible. Wash out and shampoo. Your hair will have more volume and shine!

The Incredible Egg Conditioner

My grandmother believed eggs were the single best thing for the hair. This recipe will make your hair feel incredible! Egg will not only condition your hair, but will leave it very shiny since it's high in vitamins and calcium. You'll be hooked on this easy recipe after the first time—and your hair will never look better.

INGREDIENTS

   1 teaspoon olive oil

   2 egg yolks

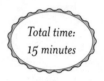

Total time:
15 minutes

Crack the eggs and separate the yolks from the whites. You will only need the yolks. (Save the egg whites for breakfast in the morning or a face mask.) Mix the olive oil and egg yolks in a small bowl. Now put the conditioner in your dry hair, starting at the scalp and working it down. Leave the mixture in for 10 minutes, then shampoo your hair. You won't believe the shine!

Babushka's Beauty Tip:

An A-list actress swears by this simple champagne rinse to work wonders on hair color: Combine 6 ounces of champagne with your regular shampoo. The tartaric acid in champagne will bring out your natural highlights or brighten any you may have added. Shampoo, rinse, and be on your way!

✳ BRING BACK BATHING CAPS! ✳

I am such a believer in bathing caps! They are highly glamorous and protect your hair! After applying color, care, and conditioner, do you really want to ruin a good head of hair? By preventing your hair from getting wet, these caps save you from that brittle grasslike hair that comes from swimming all summer long.

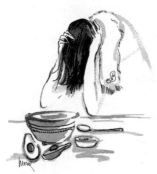

Mayo-Avocado Dip

When it comes to the hair, mayonnaise and avocado are amazing! This recipe offers a little of both. You can't imagine the amount of vitamins and minerals your hair will soak up with these two key ingredients.

INGREDIENTS

¾ cup mayonnaise

½ avocado

Total time: 35 minutes

Cut open the avocado and put half inside the blender (without the skin or pit). Add the mayo and blend for 1 minute or until creamy (with a mashed potato–like consistency). From the root down, begin massaging the mixture through the hair. Leave the conditioner in for 20 minutes and shampoo.

Forget Flyaways

Everyone hates those unforgiving flyaway hairs. It's so annoying when those ever-rebellious strands just won't get in line. In this recipe, add the ingredients below to your everyday conditioner. This is the perfect remedy to get hair to stay put.

INGREDIENTS

½ cup conditioner

¼ cup honey

1 tablespoon almond oil

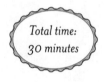

Total time:
30 minutes

Mix all the ingredients, blending well. Apply the mixture to damp hair. Work it through your hair thoroughly. Leave it on for 20 minutes and shampoo.

Babushka's Beauty Tip:

I work with an actress who has very dry hair and uses olive oil for those wild hairs. She simply pours ¼ teaspoon of olive oil into her hands, rubs them together, and lightly brushes her hair with the olive oil.

Made in the Shade

Now that your hair's in good shape, why not add a little color and shine? This isn't permanent color to cover your roots, but it will make your hair look richer. Think of it as a temporary rinse. My grandmother regularly applied tea to women's hair to give it a little oomph!

INGREDIENTS

For dark hair: two black tea bags

For blond hair: two chamomile
    tea bags

8 ounces hot water

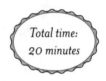

*Total time:
20 minutes*

Place the tea bags in hot water for 2 minutes. Remove the bags and let the water cool. When the tea is lukewarm, put it on your hair for 15 minutes and rinse out.

Hey, Red

INGREDIENTS

½ cup beet juice

½ cup carrot juice

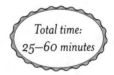

*Total time:
25–60 minutes*

Mix the ingredients together, and pour over clean, damp hair. Wrap your hair in plastic and apply a hot towel with medium dryer heat over it for 20 minutes, or sit in the sun for 30 minutes to an hour.

Babushka's Beauty Tip:

We've all had those days when we need a little color correction but don't have time to get to the salon. If you want to rejuvenate blond hair and get rid of brassy tones, tomato sauce will "lift" the color. It will also neutralize green tones.

✳ GRAY ROOTS ✳

No time for a color touch-up? Use colored mascara that matches your hair to instantly cover gray hairs until you can get to the salon. Obviously this method works best on dark hair!

Smooth Moves

This hair mask will nourish the hair and make it feel soft and healthy. Avocado is so moisturizing for the hair, as is wheat germ oil. Vitamin E strengthens the strands while cantaloupe and banana provide vital nutrients to the hair. Now throw yogurt in the mix to perfect the pH balance. I have clients who say they don't know whether to eat the mixture or put it in their hair. It will resemble a smoothie in texture and even taste!

INGREDIENTS

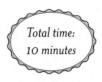

Total time:
10 minutes

½ banana

¼ cantaloupe

¼ avocado

1 tablespoon wheat germ oil

1 tablespoon yogurt

Vitamin E capsule

Blend all the ingredients in a blender on high for 1 minute. Leave the conditioner in for 8 minutes and rinse out. Follow with a good shampoo!

Baby Shampoo

My grandmother used to put this on my head when I was a baby. It was how she washed my hair. There is nothing gentler on the hair. Years later, I used the recipe on my own babies. If you have a sensitive scalp, you'll love this shampoo. I've changed the recipe a little (from regular to skim milk) but think it works brilliantly with either.

INGREDIENTS

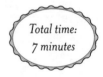

Total time:
7 minutes

1 egg

1 cup skim milk

Beat the egg and pour in the skim milk. When it all becomes foamy, rub it on your scalp. Leave it on for 5 minutes. Rinse the hair well with water.

✳ TIPS FOR YOUR TRESSES ✳

*S*ome of Hollywood's hottest hairdressers say to get beautiful hair, follow these simple rules:

1. Wash your hair on a night you aren't going out. Let it dry naturally so as not to do another night of damage from the blow dryer. Hair also looks better at least 12 to 24 hours after a washing, since it gets back some of the natural oils.

2. When using a blow dryer, don't have the setting on hot since it can be very damaging to the hair.

3. Try to avoid hair gels and other products with alcohol since they dry out hair.

4. Shower with warm water. Hot water can dry the scalp.

5. Apply wheat germ oil to your hair regularly. It's incredible for conditioning the hair.

6. Protect your hair anytime you go in saltwater or chlorine.

Oil Out

Adding just a little aloe and lemon to your daily shampoo will help eliminate oil. It can't be easier!

INGREDIENTS

    I teaspoon aloe vera gel

    I tablespoon fresh lemon juice

    ¼ cup any shampoo

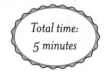

Total time:
5 minutes

Combine the ingredients in a small bowl or a cup. Stir and apply to your hair. Leave on for 2 minutes, and this mixture will wash the excess oil out of your hair.

Dry Hair Eraser

Who doesn't love the blow dryer or flat iron? But let's get real—both of these wonderful tools can make hair rather dry. This recipe will add a little moisture and make your hair smell great! There's nothing worse than brittle or dry hair, but it's really an easy issue to combat.

INGREDIENTS

Total time:
5 minutes

    1 teaspoon lavender oil

    1 teaspoon coconut milk

Combine ingredients when your hair is dry. Massage the mixture through before bed. (I always put down a towel on my pillow before going to sleep with this mixture on.) When you get up in the morning, simply rinse it out. You won't believe the texture of your hair!

✳ DANDRUFF REMEDY ✳

To combat dandruff, simply add 2 crushed aspirins in your normal shampoo. Expensive dandruff shampoo contains salicylic acid, which is present in aspirin, so it works in the same way. It will act quickly to clear your scalp of dandruff and grime at a fraction of the cost.

Coconut Delight

This is an easy way to get shampoo and conditioner in one. You can add it to your favorite shampoo. I suggest using almond oil, but if you can get your hands on avocado oil, use it!

INGREDIENTS

Total time: 5 minutes

    2 teaspoons almond oil

    1½ tablespoon coconut milk

    ¼ cup shampoo of your choice

This mixture should be enough for one to three shampoos (depending on how long and thick the hair). Combine the ingredients in a bowl and whisk together for 2–3 minutes. You can store it in the bathroom (no need to put in the refrigerator). Shake well before each use.

Cider Conditioner (for Dry Hair)

This recipe is perfect for people with dry or damaged hair since it's a pretty heavy-duty conditioner. When the layer of oil in the hair is broken down, the moisture trapped below evaporates, leaving the hair to dry out and become more prone to damage. It isn't long before you end up with dry, unmanageable areas, complete with split ends and broken shafts. This conditioner will help.

INGREDIENTS

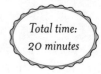

Total time: 20 minutes

    2 teaspoons sesame oil

    1½ teaspoons coconut oil

    2 teaspoons honey

    1 teaspoon cider vinegar

Pour the sesame oil and coconut oil into a small saucepan. Warm it over low heat (do not boil). Remove the pan from the heat and stir in the honey and vinegar. While it's warm, use this mixture on your hair after you shampoo. Leave it on for 15 minutes before rinsing it off with warm water. The results? Healthy hair!

✳ BEER, BABY ✳

Did you know beer can...

1. **Highlight your hair.** Soak your hair in beer and then sit in the sun. It will bring out any natural highlights.

2. **Fix any out-of-place hairs on your head or even eyebrows.** It has hairspray-like qualities as it is sticky enough to restrain any displaced hairs that you might catch in the mirror.

3. **Be used in a bath.** Now this is really going through a six-pack! You can use a dark beer in your bath. Add two bottles of dark beer to your bathwater and the yeast will soften and soothe your skin.

4. **Soothe those tired feet.** Pour a few cold bottles of beer into a bucket and allow the carbonation and temperature to go to work.

5. **Shine your gold jewelry (without stones).** Simply pour some beer into a soft cloth and wipe the jewelry down gently until it's dry. This will polish your gold and give it some extra shine.

6. **Marinate meat!** It is brilliant for the weekend BBQ!

Chapter Nine

Take It Off

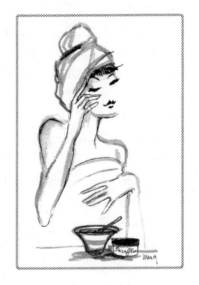

My grandmother would often joke that God made her half man by giving her a mustache. In her fifties, those unsightly hairs on her chin began surfacing. This was one of those rare beauty problems that drove her insane. Back then we thought it was kind of funny. But when I was scratching my chin on a date recently and felt a little hair, I wondered if it wasn't a little bit of karma coming my way. Thank goodness for tweezers, laser hair removal, and wax!

Many women suffer from unwanted facial hair and it isn't fun! According to one study, approximately 20 million American women remove facial hair at least once a week. From chins to upper lips to eyebrows—facial hair maintenance is a chore.

Now, add insult to injury and throw in the bikini wax. Ouch! There's no doubt hair grows back slower with a wax since you're pulling it from the root. Depending on the person, hair will usually start growing back in a week or two after a good wax. You can save money by waxing at home (but don't do the eyebrows)!

This chapter tackles all those hair-raising issues—and those girly questions like what to do about ingrown hairs or if it's best to wax, shave, or pluck. There are a number of great recipes offering up everything from shaving cream to potions for ingrown hairs.

And remember, you can't catch a cold from being in the snow, nor do hairs grow back thicker after you pluck them. I promise. In fact, it's quite the opposite. Repeatedly plucking hairs can scar the hair follicle, which over time can lead to permanent loss. Talk about saving money!

WAXING AT HOME

Doing your own facial waxing is pretty easy (the bikini area is not as easy), but before you get going, make sure to stock up on all the essentials:

✳ **Wax.** I prefer creamy wax rather than the clear stuff.
✳ **Baby powder.** The area in question needs to be dry.

✳ **Wooden sticks.** These applicators are available at most beauty supply stores. Or try an old Popsicle stick or the other end of an old spatula.

✳ **Olive oil and ice.** Use these to remove wax from the body or clothing. (You don't want to get it on clothing or furniture. It's tough to get off!)

✳ **Aloe-based gel, sour cream, or buttermilk (all very soothing after waxing).** It will bring down bumps and redness.

✳ **Tweezers (for ingrown hairs or anything you miss).**

✳ **Waxing strips.** Or you can simply cut up an old cotton T-shirt into 3 by 5 strips. It's a good way to recycle an old T-shirt and they work really well.

How to get the best wax:

✳ Pull or pin your hair back. You don't want wax in your hair. It's worse than gum.

✳ Put baby powder on the area you want to wax (upper lip, chin, bikini line, legs, or underarms).

✳ Heat wax. You want one that can be zapped in a microwave.

✳ Apply the wax to the area, but don't put it on too thick or it's impossible to pull off.

✳ Place the strip on top of the wax and smooth it in the direction of the hair growth, but leave two inches at the end so it's easy to grab and pull. Press your finger firmly over the strip.

✳ Take a deep breath and pull it off.

✳ Everyone will miss a hair or two. Go back and clean up with the tweezers.

✳ If you have bumps or redness, apply aloe. Aloe is best on the face while sour cream or buttermilk is fabulous on the legs and bikini line.

✳ If you notice a little patch of wax later that didn't come off, put a little olive oil on the area and it should slip right off. If that doesn't work, apply ice and it should harden and peel away.

A Word of Warning about Eyebrows

If you're doing your own brows, don't use wax! Half my business is shaping brows and I can't tell you how many clients come in with eyebrow emergencies after trying to wax their own at home. It's so easy to make a little mistake, but on an eyebrow it becomes impossible to hide.

As you can imagine, it isn't fun to wait for hair to grow back. So here's what you need to do: Pluck the brows at home rather than wax. Eyebrows are important since they frame the eyes. They can either lift or bring down your eyes, so it's crucial to get it right! I prefer a brow that looks fuller rather than too thin. Thin brows are aging and can create a hard, angry look. Thicker brows, on the other hand, tend to create a softer, more youthful look.

⚬〜〜 SHAVING 〜〜⚬

My grandmother always used a razor for hair removal. After all, there weren't so many options back then. Because of my babushka, there is a sentimental side of me that has a soft spot for shaving. Shaving often gets a bad rap. Shaving will bring hair back in a couple of days because the hair is cut at skin level. It will also grow back coarser because of the angle. Eventually if you let the hair continue to grow, it will soften up. But who wants to wait that long?

Still, when it comes to legs, sometimes shaving is just easier on a daily basis.

Here's the best way to get a good shave:

   1. You don't want to shave dry skin. Shaving is a natural exfoliant and you'll clog up the razor with dead skin while putting yourself at risk for nicks.

   2. There's no need to waste your money on shaving creams formulated especially for women. They are virtually the same as the creams sold for men.

   3. Don't forget to exfoliate before shaving. It gets rid of all the dead skin cells that could clog up your razor, preventing a close shave.

   4. Since your leg hairs grow down, you'll want to start at your ankles and shave up. For underarms, shave in every direction since the hair there grows every which way.

5. When finished shaving, apply oil or moisturizer. The skin on your legs has few oil glands and has a tendency for dryness.

How Much Do We Detest Ingrown Hairs?

Let me just say it's tough being a woman! Sometimes maintenance is a full-time job. As if a bikini wax weren't painful enough, there's the ever-annoying problem of ingrown hairs! When the hair grows back, since it's curly and course, it can get stuck underneath the skin, causing ingrown hairs. Sometimes you may need to get rid of an ingrown hair if it becomes too painful. Use a pair of sterile tweezers with some rubbing alcohol, and pluck the hair out. Wipe the area with some alcohol afterward.

Another treatment that works is to put witch hazel on the area if it looks a little infected. To treat ingrown hairs that have become really inflamed, use hot and cold compresses. The following are a few good remedies for ingrown hairs as well.

Soak It in Sugar

This is the first line of defense against ingrown hairs. Exfoliation is crucial. For women, the worst place for ingrown hairs is along the bikini line. Getting rid of ingrown hairs can be quite painful. This recipe will relieve the pain. It's perfect as a preventive tool as well.

INGREDIENTS

¾ cup sugar

½ tablespoon fresh lemon juice

Total time:
10 minutes

Take It Off

  1½ tablespoon cornstarch

  3 tablespoons honey

  2 tablespoon apple cider vinegar

Combine the ingredients in a bowl and stir well. Lightly dust a little flour on the skin around the ingrown hair—it will soak up the excess oil on the surface of the skin. Now scrub the mixture for about 5 minutes directly on the ingrown hairs and let it sit for a few minutes. Rinse off with warm water.

Sweet Scrubs

Here are two more fantastic remedies for ingrown hairs. This is one of the few times when you can indulge in sugar without all the guilt that usually goes along with it. So go for it!

INGREDIENTS

  1 cup sugar

  ½ cup olive oil

  3 drops vanilla

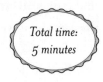

Total time:
5 minutes

Mix the ingredients together and scrub all over the areas where there are ingrown hairs.

This next one is even easier . . .

  ¼ cup moisturizer (I love Eucerin.)

  2 tablespoons sugar

Again rub on any area where you have ingrown hairs. These are also both fantastic on the feet and hands. Make sure you rinse off the scrub thoroughly.

The Ingrown Headache

Remember, honey is a natural antiseptic and moisturizer. The aspirin (don't use it if you're allergic) will reduce swelling. And the oil will moisturize and hopefully take away some of the redness. This is a quick cure for ingrown hairs.

INGREDIENTS

Total time:
20 minutes

1 teaspoon honey

½ tablespoon olive oil

3 uncoated aspirin tablets

Place the honey and olive oil in the microwave for 10 seconds (or until it softens up a bit). Using a fork, crush up the aspirin as well as you can. Throw in the finely crushed aspirin and stir the concoction together. The consistency will be a little strange but it works! Apply to the infected areas and leave on for 10–15 minutes. Wash it off with lukewarm water.

Babushka's Beauty Tip:

To reduce redness after a bikini wax or shaving, try a little sour cream, which will cool down the area. My grandmother loved sour cream to treat any kind of irritation.

Shaving Oil

Try using this oil to shave and you'll never go back to cream. You won't believe how fantastic your legs will look and feel. My grandmother used sunflower oil to shave her legs and thought it was the best product ever. With the recipe below, your legs will look gorgeous!

INGREDIENTS

Total time:
10 minutes

 3 ounces almond oil

 ½ ounce sesame oil

 ½ ounce canola oil

 ½ ounce wheat germ oil

Get a small bowl and throw in all the ingredients. Stir and put the mixture in an old bottle. Whenever you want to use it, just shake it up for a few minutes and throw it on, then shave. You'll love the results!

Shaving Cream

Many people prefer to use shaving cream so I'm offering this recipe. It's really quite simple though it will take a little time in the cooking and setting of the cream. You can add one drop of an essential oil after you take it off the stove if you'd like some kind of scent. I suggest lavender.

INGREDIENTS

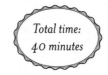

Total time:
40 minutes

 1 teaspoon sunflower oil

 ½ cup unscented glycerin soap

In a double boiler, cut the glycerin soap up into small pieces. Quickly stir in the sunflower oil and move from the double boiler into a small bowl. The mixture should set very quickly.

Simply wet a shaving brush with warm water and rub the soap until it begins to lather. Apply it to the legs and start shaving.

Babushka's Beauty Tip:

Hair conditioner is also a great substitute if you ever run out of shaving cream. It can actually be great on the legs. Just slather on the conditioner and you're good to go.

Chapter Ten

Hands and Feet

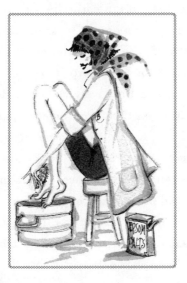

$\mathcal{M}$y babushka always believed a woman should never feel compelled to reveal her age: It's her private information and she can choose whether or not to disclose it. After all, you're only as old as you look and feel. Women come into my salon all the time and I think they're thirty-five when they are almost fifty! I've also seen the opposite, too—girls in their twenties who live a bit too hard and look much older.

Most of us concentrate on keeping our face, legs, arms, and stomach in good shape but neglect some key areas. Don't forget about the hands and feet! They can be a dead giveaway as to a person's true age. My babushka believed if a woman took care of her feet, they could always look soft and young. With all the open-toe shoes and sandals, feet are often out on display—so take care of those tootsies.

One way to do this is to slather petroleum jelly all over the feet and throw on a pair of socks before going to bed. Your feet will feel fabulous in the morning! One other piece of information I'd like to impart is this: Don't go barefoot! There's nothing rougher on the feet. I know it feels good, but please throw on some slippers or shoes!

Hands are also a dead giveaway as to a woman's age! We can't forget about the ever-important hands. And that's because along with the face, your hands are one of the most exposed parts of the body.

Not only do we put our hands through the rigors of daily work, but they're also exposed to damaging environmental influences, such as sun and dry weather. It's important to take preventive measures to ward off signs of premature aging.

The recipes in this chapter will demonstrate easy ways to get rid of dry skin and pamper the feet and hands.

HANDS

I've worked with some great manicurists and all agree it's important to take good care of the hands. Keeping them soft and smooth is easy with a little weekly tender loving care. I have a simple test you can do at home to see if your hands are in need of some TLC:

✳ Scratch the skin on the top of your hands. If you see lines and wrinkles, you need to moisturize and exfoliate.

✳ If you pinch the skin on your hands and let go and it doesn't return to the original position immediately, your hands are too dry.

I must confess there are times I've failed both. But when I'm diligent about caring for my hands, I can easily pass the test. Here's a handful of information to help:

1. **Moisturize hands after washing.** Soap can be so drying. I wash my hands at least ten times a day but always use some kind of very rich moisturizer directly after. Many times it's just olive oil.

2. **Don't forget gloves.** Wear gloves in cold weather or when washing dishes—obviously not the same type.

3. **Treat your hands at night.** If my hands are looking really dry, I often coat them in petroleum jelly and then put them in socks. You can't believe the difference in the morning. It really works!

4. **Use sunscreen.** Just as you'd use sunscreen every day for your face, do the same with your hands, neck, arms, or any other place exposed to the sun.

5. **Pamper your hands as you'd pamper your face.** If you like to use certain creams and potions on your face, throw it on your hands as well. I have

a client who uses glycolic products on her face, hands, and feet.

6. **Soak your cuticles and nails.** Keeping your nails healthy will help the hands stay looking young.

Soaking cuticles in egg yolks works quite well since they contain biotin, a B vitamin. A couple times a week you can put your nails (for 5 minutes) in walnut oil or almond oil. Or try a mayo bath every couple of weeks. Get a small bowl full of mayo and soak your nails for 10 minutes.

The 10-Minute Manicure

* File your nails while they're completely dry. You'll get a better shape.
* To keep hands moist and smooth, I like to use a little scrub made of 2 tablespoons of brown sugar and 3 tablespoons of olive oil. (There are other great scrubs in this chapter as well.) Scrub your hands and push back the cuticles with a toothbrush or Popsicle stick. My grandmother never believed in cutting the cuticles because, when you do so, you get more dead skin.
* Rinse with warm water and pat dry.
* Apply nail polish, sweeping on polish the way they do in salons from base to tip.

Gently place olive oil carefully on each nail 30 minutes after the manicure. It will speed up the drying process and avoid drying out your nails.

Hands like Honey

This is a recipe designed to soften and moisturize the skin. It's like nothing you've ever tried before. The four ingredients all work well together. In this scrub there's a little bit of everything for the hands. My grandmother came up with this recipe but I changed sunflower oil to walnut oil. She also used a different grain, but I love oatmeal.

INGREDIENTS

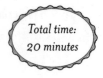

Total time:
20 minutes

½ cup honey
½ cup lemon juice
1 cup almond oil
1 cup oatmeal

Combine all the ingredients in a mixing bowl. Stir together and toss into a food processor or blender. Blend for about 2 minutes. Apply to the hands and keep on for 15 minutes (with a towel under them). Rinse with lukewarm water.

The Yellowing Effect

Have you ever noticed how your nails may look yellow after you first remove nail polish? It probably happens more often when using darker nail colors such as deep reds. Don't fret—the nails are usually yellow because they're stained, possibly from tobacco if you're a smoker. There are a number of natural ways to whiten your nails.

1. Soak your nails in an equal mixture of lemon juice and water for 5 minutes.

2. Put whitening toothpaste on an old toothbrush and clean your nails.

3. Mix 1 tablespoon of hydrogen peroxide with 2 tablespoons of baking soda. Put this paste under and across each nail and sit with the solution on for 3 minutes.

4. To prevent the yellowing effect, always put on a base coat so those dark colors won't stain your nails in the first place.

STILETTOS SUFFERERS

Nothing gets between me and my stilettos. I love wearing high heels, and there is nothing like a fabulous pair of Manolos! If you're anything like me, you love stilettos, too! Fashionable shoes are fun but not always the most comfortable. In the name of fashion, I'm willing to suffer. But there are ways to make moving in heels a little easier.

After a long night in heels, the feet can get sore. So as not to retire the stilettos (even for one night), I suggest the following for taking care of sore feet:

1. Slather Vicks VapoRub all over your feet and throw on a pair of socks before bed. Your feet will feel incredible in the morning!

2. Soak the feet for 10 minutes in sugarless carbonated water.

3. Put 2 tablespoons of Epsom salt into water and soak your feet for 10 minutes.

Soothing Stilettos

My grandmother never wore high heels but I know she would have approved of others wearing them. There is nothing more feminine than a heel on a woman's foot. Listen, I'm not saying wear high heels even if it's going to kill your feet! This next recipe is for the girl who just needs a little relief after having to walk too far in stilettos—something I don't highly recommend!

1 tablespoon olive oil

1 teaspoon aloe vera

1 teaspoon wheat germ

5 drops eucalyptus

1 tablespoon mineral water

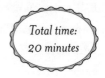

Total time:
20 minutes

In a medium-sized bowl, mix together all the ingredients. Soak your feet for 10 minutes and then moisturize.

Babushka's Beauty Tip:

After a soak, I like to slather petroleum jelly on my feet and then slip on a pair of socks. Your feet will be so soft and smooth the next morning.

Clear Away Calluses

The best way to remove calluses is to use products containing salicylic acid. But did you know most dandruff shampoos also contain salicylic acid? It could be in your home—just look on the back of the bottle for that vital ingredient. If you are suffering from calluses, simply rub the dandruff shampoo on your feet for 5 minutes, then wash it off. It can be extremely drying so don't forget to apply olive oil afterward. Follow it up with a little salt and soda. This next recipe will also help those calluses.

INGREDIENTS
   ½ cup baking soda
   ½ cup kosher salt
   1 loofah

Total time:
25 minutes

Fill a big pan or bowl (large enough for your feet) with warm water. Throw in the baking soda and kosher salt and stir. Soak your feet for 20 minutes, then scrub the callus or corn with the loofah. What a difference a little salt and soda make!

Strawberry Scrub

As you know, the skin on your hands and feet needs to be exfoliated and renewed just like any other part of the body. I can't live without my scrubs and homemade scented oils. This is one way in which I really love to pamper myself. I adore this scrub and so does my daughter! My babushka loved it as well. She used sunflower oil, but I've changed it to olive oil. One year on my birthday, she mixed up the scrub and did an

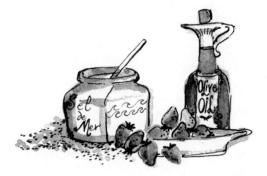

evening of pampering with my favorite meal of tomatoes and sauer-kraut. Strawberries were the dessert!

INGREDIENTS

9 strawberries

2 tablespoons olive oil

1 teaspoon sea salt

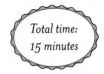

Total time: 15 minutes

Mix all the ingredients in a blender on high for about 2 minutes. Now massage into the hands and feet for 10 minutes. Rinse it off and pat dry. Strawberries contain a natural fruit acid that is fantastic for exfoliating.

Sweet and Salty Scrub

This recipe is great for getting rid of dead skin that seems to just hang on to the heels of the feet. Whenever doing pedicures at home, this is a must! Salt and sugar both work quite well to remove dead skin, as does the cornmeal and oatmeal. Now throw in a little moisturizer and your feet are standing pretty!

INGREDIENTS

> ¼ cup sea salt
>
> 1 tablespoon sugar
>
> ¼ cup oatmeal (Grind it in a blender before throwing it in the mix.)
>
> ¼ cup cornmeal
>
> 2 tablespoons aloe vera gel
>
> ¼ cup unscented body lotion (You know I like Eucerin.)

Total time: 15 minutes

As you mix all the ingredients together, it will form a thick paste. Massage into your feet and give them a good scrub for as long as possible.

The Perfect Pedicure

It's very important that a woman's feet always look fabulous! Like a manicure, a pedicure is also pretty easy to do at home. Ideally you want to use a huge pan (reserved solely for pedicures) to soak your feet.

✳ Remove old polish with a cotton ball.

✳ Fill up your pan with enough warm water to soak your feet and then add some Epsom salt and 2 tablespoons of vanilla. Or you can get fancy and add flower petals.

✳ Dry your feet with a clean towel.

✳ Clip your toenails back with a nail clipper. (I personally prefer very short toenails.) Now whip out the nail file and do a little shaping.

* Exfoliate! I have some good scrubs in this chapter. Pick one out and get going!

* Moisturize. Massage your feet and legs with a rich cream. (I love Eucerin. It's moisturizing and unscented.)

* Soften. Add a little olive oil to the feet to soften and revitalize rough areas.

* Push back the cuticles using tweezers or a Popsicle stick.

* Polish the nails. Apply a base coat first and then two coats, followed by a top coat.

* Take out that olive oil again. After nails have been drying for an hour, place a drop on each nail to aid in the process.

Babushka's Beauty Tip:

If you suddenly need to run out of the house or a nail salon, I have the perfect solution! Fifteen minutes after a pedicure, put a drop of olive oil on each toenail and place plastic wrap around the toes. Make sure they are all covered. Now put on your socks, tennis shoes, or boots and your toenails shouldn't smudge. I've done it a number of times. In the middle of winter in New York it seems every nail salon has plastic wrap and oil for this very reason.

Chapter Eleven

Buff the Body

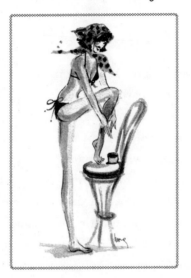

Don't be scared off by the title of this chapter. I'm not going to make you run off to the gym, but rather let you know ways to beat the system. In other words, this chapter is about camouflage. It's filled with recipes to help reduce the appearance of cellulite and make your body glow.

My grandmother didn't understand why any woman would want to be skinny. She thought a woman's body should be full and favored the classic hourglass figure. Her famous saying was, "When a woman is too skinny, men won't want her. Man is not a dog," she would bark upon seeing a thin woman. "They won't jump on a bone."

She would be appalled today to see women obsess over their weight. Trust me, she'd think I was a bag of bones.

Where we would agree is on a woman staying in good physical shape and having a tanned and toned body.

SUN-KISSED

The sun-kissed look became chic in the 1920s when style icon Coco Chanel paraded around fashion shows with a bronze tan following a Mediterranean vacation. After that, suntans suddenly became a status symbol.

This love affair with the sun would continue for a number of decades—until eventually skin experts set sun lovers straight. However, the damaging news about tanning created new opportunities for cosmetic companies. Today spray tans and bronzers are all the rage.

But they don't come without their own set of problems. Clients frequently ask how to get rid of those sun streaks from self-tanners. The good news—it isn't permanent. Bronzers in a bottle will begin to fade in a few days, but if you need an immediate fix for a particular occasion, there is a solution.

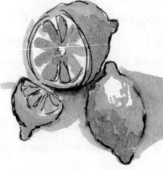

Here are four ways to tone down that tan:

✳ Apply lemon juice on your body and it will start to lighten up the self-tanner.

✳ My favorite, vodka, will also begin erasing that bad tan!

✳ Place baking soda on a wet washcloth and then apply it on the splotches. It will exfoliate skin and act as a sort of bleach.

✳ For too much color under the fingernails, hands, toe-nails, and feet, you can apply facial bleach for about 10 minutes. Or simply put some hydrogen peroxide on those areas and get the color to fade.

The following are tips on applying a self-tanner properly:

✳ Take a shower and always exfoliate first since it will allow for a more even distribution.

✳ Wear gloves. My clients are split as to whether gloves help apply a more even self-tanner. But there is nothing worse than having orange hands!

✳ Squeeze the self-tanner out of the tube and onto your hands. I usually begin with my legs and work up.

✳ Don't forget the feet and go all around the toes! But don't be heavy-handed in these areas since they can get too dark very quickly.

✳ Don't overdo the knees and elbows since self-tanners can soak up in those areas and make them appear dirty rather than sun-kissed.

✳ Work quickly in a circular motion to avoid streaks. Moving it up and down will ensure streaking! Don't!

✳ Work your way up the entire body the same way.

✳ You should now proudly be touting a streak-free tan!

CELLULITE

No body is perfect. In fact, can we bond over the fact that every woman has cellulite? Even some of the thinnest models have it, but these glamazons are fortunate enough to work in an age of computer technology so everything looks smooth in their photos. If only we could create those effects in real life.

I always think Europeans are more comfortable in their own skin than Americans. Go to beaches in the South of France and heavy women with saggy breasts and cellulite are baring it all, right next to the stick-thin model! I'm always surprised but think, "Good for them." No one really cares. It's all in our head.

So let's look at the facts. There is no real cure for cellulite. So why do many treatments appear to work for a bit? Because cellulite is fat that is dimpled close to the surface of the skin, any treatment that pushes that fat deeper into the skin will temporarily improve the appearance of cellulite. That's fine if you just need to get into a bathing suit for a day or so and need a temporary fix. Just know it won't go away forever.

There are ways to make our bodies and our skin look

the best they can. The following are some good recipes for the body.

Oat Couture

This is the perfect body scrub to use before getting into a bathing suit. Why not have the skin look silky and smooth to boost your confidence? So much of looking good in a bathing suit is the skin looking nice. If you want to use this recipe all over the body, simply triple it.

INGREDIENTS

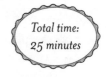

Total time: 25 minutes

    2 tablespoons rolled oats, ground

    2 teaspoons brown sugar

    2 tablespoons aloe vera

    1 teaspoon lemon juice

Put the rolled oats in the blender and grind into a very fine powder. Place the powder in a small mixing bowl. Add the brown sugar and lemon juice. Mix well. Now add the aloe vera and stir to form a paste. Be sure there are no lumps. Dampen the skin and massage the paste onto it. Rinse with warm water.

Mustard Body Wrap

Here's a good recipe to smooth out the thigh area for 24 hours. It's basically a way to reduce the appearance of cellulite. It isn't a permanent solution but it does get the blood circulating all over the tops of the legs. Personally, I love it before jumping into a bathing suit or a tight skirt or dress. You definitely need a little time and a place to relax while this recipe kicks in. My clients call it one of my crazy Ukrainian recipes. I simply love it and do it a couple times a year!

INGREDIENTS

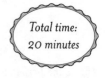

Total time:
20 minutes

2 tablespoons spicy mustard

2 tablespoons vodka

Mix up the mustard and vodka and massage it onto the tops of the legs. Then cover the area with plastic wrap. If you want to take an extra step, simply get in bed and put a blanket over you to heat up the body. After 15 minutes, remove the plastic and wash off the mixture.

GLITTER AND TANNERS

Body Glitter

When you're on vacation and want to throw on that sexy dress, why not add a little body glitter to go with it. Body glitter can even dress up a tank top and shorts. I do this sometimes with my daughter and her friends. They love it — it's just one of those frivolous girl things! We like throwing in a little gold — especially with a tan. Talk about bringing a shimmer to the skin!

INGREDIENTS

Total time:
10 minutes

3 tablespoons aloe vera gel

1 teaspoon very fine glitter (any color)

1 drop lavender essential oil

Add as much glitter to the aloe vera gel as you want. I always start with less and test it out until I like the mixture. It's optional to add essential oil. Store any unused portion in an old glass container at room temperature. You'll love this body glitter—it's so fun!

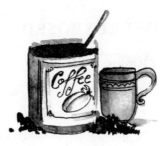

Coffee Tanner

A tan is the best camouflage for cellulite, but who knew coffee grounds could give your skin such a glow? Talk about recycling! So don't throw out those used grounds. This coffee scrub is easy but I won't deny it can be quite messy! I like doing this in an empty bathtub or a shower. I often suggest using a body scrub before applying this one.

INGREDIENTS

Total time:
20 minutes

1 cup warm used coffee grounds
2 tablespoons olive oil

Combine the olive oil and coffee grounds. Apply them on your legs, arms, face, or wherever else you want a little color. Keep on the body for 15 minutes, then wash off. Your skin will have that perfect glow! This coffee recipe has taken Hollywood by storm. My babushka would have been shocked! It's funny that her old Ukrainian recipe is a must-have for a number of actresses before hitting the red carpet. Not only does it add a golden touch but it makes the skin soft and smooth.

OVEREXPOSED

Sunburn Soother

There's nothing worse than hitting the beach and realizing at the end of the day you've simply overdone it. Your shoulders are sore to the touch, and your legs are burning up. It's impossible to get comfortable, much less get a good night's sleep. But help is on the way from the ever-magical aloe plant. This will reduce the pain and peeling. Aloe is very effective at relieving pain and inflammation. The next two recipes will save your sunburned skin!

INGREDIENTS

Total time: 5 minutes

    1 cup aloe vera juice

    1–2 drops lavender essential oil

    1 hard plastic spray bottle

Pour the aloe and the lavender in the bottle and mix well. Gently spray on sunburned skin as needed!

INGREDIENTS

    ½ cup aloe vera gel

    1 tablespoon chamomile flowers (or open a
        chamomile tea bag)

    2 tablespoons vitamin E oil

Mix all the ingredients together and apply to the sunburned area. This recipe also hydrates and moisturizes dry skin.

Burnout

This is a very old-fashioned recipe we used in the Ukraine on one of those rare occasions we'd actually get sunburned. (Of course, it seemed like the sun was never out.) Since moving to the States, I've had to use this recipe a number of times because I didn't realize how quickly the skin could get burned even with sunscreen.

INGREDIENTS

Total time: 35 minutes

7 tablespoons buttermilk

3 tablespoons tomato juice

Put the ingredients into a small bowl and mix well. Apply to sunburned areas and wash off after about 30 minutes. Repeat every few hours. Put on this remedy until the sunburn cools down.

Babushka's Beauty Tip:

Did you know that simply applying sour cream to a sunburn does wonders? It is so soothing and you'll appreciate the relief it brings.

Chapter Twelve

~~~~~~~~~~

Doing the Decades

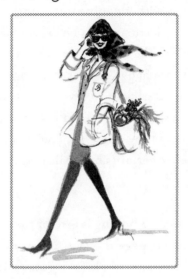

*M*y grandmother believed skin should (and could) glow at any age. I know it's possible because in the worst circumstances (cold weather and little money) she was able to produce incredible results on women of all ages. She didn't believe one remedy worked on everyone— her recipes were designed for a particular person with her age in mind.

What we worry about in our twenties (oily skin and acne) isn't necessarily an issue in our forties. Since every decade poses different problems, this chapter is designed as a sort of play-by-play of what to do at different times in your life. But with women looking so great at every age, the rules continue to change. Old rules were: You shouldn't have long hair past forty. Wrong! You shouldn't wear a short skirt past forty. Wrong again! But there is a way to dress sexy without going too young.

Enough of my lecturing—time to get to the good stuff. First, let's look at the various elements that will age us too quickly—those habits such as smoking, sunning, and staying out too late. Hate to say it, but taken to excess, these are no-no's for all ages! I'm not saying you have to live a totally clean life—come on, you've got to have some fun. But there are certain chemicals that can be toxic and very aging.

1. **Smoking.** Smoking is bad for the entire body and can seriously age the face. Have you ever seen the lines around a smoker's mouth? Have I said enough?

2. **Sun.** I love the way a suntan looks. Anytime the sun was shining, my grandmother would get us out in the early morning or late afternoon. Back then we didn't wear sunscreen but I do now. While I know vitamin D is crucial, there are times and ways to soak in that D while still protecting your skin.

3. **Drinking alcohol.** Smoking and drinking dehydrate the skin. That said, I do like my vodka. But after a night of drinking, I take in tons of water.

4. Lack of sleep. My grandmother always thought women should sleep exactly seven hours a night—no more and no less (I personally believe eight hours is ideal!).

5. Yo-yo dieting. The other bad habit is yo-yo dieting. When our weight goes up and down too much, it can take its toll on the skin.

TEENS AND TWENTIES

The biggest problems people face in their teens and twenties are oily skin, acne, and future sun damage. Since wrinkles aren't a big concern when you're in your twenties, why not soak up the sun? Well, the damage you do today will show up years down the road. So protect the skin now and use sunscreen all over.

Before I give out a few remedies for acne, let me start by debunking some common myths about it.

1. Sweating makes acne worse: Wrong! In fact, Stanford and Harvard did a study with three sets of teens for two weeks to look into this theory. One group didn't exercise. One group did and then immediately showered. The third group waited four hours to shower after exercising. Guess what? It didn't make a difference. (But in my experience I would suggest showering after a heavy workout.)

2. Bad acne is caused by greasy foods and chocolate: Wrong! This is one of the oldest myths out there, but scientific studies simply don't back it up. No matter how much chocolate, french fries, greasy burgers, and cheese you consume, it won't cause acne. So go for it—have that candy bar and chocolate shake, too! We can tackle acne separately.

3. Acne is only a problem when you're a teen-ager or in your twenties: Wrong! If only it were true! I have plenty of clients who get pimples in their thirties and even forties. My babushka always said, "Life isn't always fair."

4. Acne is caused by dirty skin: Wrong! No matter how often you wash your face, you can still have bad acne. While washing the face is very important, pimples start from below the skin's surface.

5. Makeup causes acne: Wrong! Even oil-based foundation doesn't cause acne.

6. The sun will burn off acne: Wrong! Sun exposure will only cause wrinkles in your future.

7. It's better to pop a pimple and get the pus out. The truth is, even though it feels really good to release the pus, a lot of it just goes in deeper. This causes more inflammation, which can lead to scarring and spread under the skin.

Acne Away

With the help of a magnifying mirror, we all like to perform major surgery—don't! It can create bad scarring.

The treatments below will aid in the battle against the ever-annoying acne.

Acne is one of the most embarrassing and difficult problems to deal with. A number of hard-core medications exist to treat acne but natural remedies can be quite effective as well. These next two recipes will help clear up skin.

Milk and Mustard

INGREDIENTS

> 1 teaspoon mustard
>
> 1 teaspoon milk

Total time: 2 minutes

Mix the ingredients together and apply to the affected areas.

Pimple Potion

INGREDIENTS

> 1 teaspoon baking soda
>
> 1 teaspoon lemon juice

Total time: 2 minutes

Mix the ingredients together and apply to the affected areas. It's a brilliant recipe for drying up pimples!

Oil Out

To fight oily skin, give this next recipe a try. Lemon is good for cleaning and getting rid of dark spots. Grapes not only are a fantastic antioxidant but will soften the skin as well. And egg whites will firm up the face! These three ingredients together will do a number on your face, including removing excess oil from your skin naturally.

INGREDIENTS

> 5 green grapes
> 1 tablespoon fresh lemon juice
> 2 egg whites
> 3 tablespoons mineral water

Total time: 25 minutes

Squeeze the juice from the grapes into a small bowl. Then throw in the lemon and egg whites. Mix well. Apply all over the face and let sit for 20 minutes.

WARNING: Egg whites will make the skin feel tight. Wash off with lukewarm water and use a cotton ball to apply mineral water all over the face.

Babushka's Beauty Tip:

For oily skin, rub on some plain milk of magnesia and let it dry. Then rinse with lukewarm water. It absorbs oil wonderfully! There are a number of actresses who use this method to reduce oil before going under strong lights.

THIRTY-SOMETHING

Bring on the changes. This is the time when most women start thinking seriously about their skin. In our thirties, fine lines and wrinkles start to creep up. I remember for the first time worrying about wrinkles when I was examining my skin under a magnifying mirror. It's not such doom and gloom. Come on, these days women are dating men ten to twenty years younger.

Here's the story: From our twenties to thirties, there is a dramatic change in how often the skin exfoliates. That means it's important to do it yourself. I promise to make it as painless as possible. A quick way to exfoliate is to make a paste with a tablespoon of cornmeal and a tablespoon of water and apply it to your skin. Use a circular motion to scrub. Make exfoliation a daily habit.

Use gentle products, moisturizer, sunscreen, vitamin C serums, and alpha hydroxy acids. Focus on damage prevention. No need for antiwrinkle masks; just protect your skin. These next recipes offer ways to take your skin from dull to dashing, as well as other treatments to protect your precious skin!

From Dull to Dashing

In your thirties, there are times you may notice your skin looking a little dull. But you can easily go from dull to dashing! Who wouldn't want to? The mixture of strawberries, oatmeal, and honey will surprise you. This recipe will give your skin a little lift.

Total time:
20 minutes

INGREDIENTS

½ cup fresh strawberries

1 tablespoon oatmeal

¼ teaspoon honey

Mix all the ingredients in a blender on high for 1 minute. The mixture should come out looking like a smoothie (although the oatmeal may make it a little lumpy). Apply all over the face and let sit for 15 minutes. Wash off with warm water and apply a moisturizer.

The C-Fusion

This is one of the best recipes for whitening and delivers a heavy dose of vitamin C to the skin. If you're having one of those days where you feel like your skin is looking dull, then this is the ideal prescription. My clients rave about this potion.

INGREDIENTS

Total time:
20 minutes

½ cup plain yogurt

1 teaspoon lemon juice

1 teaspoon lime juice

1 teaspoon grapefruit juice

1 teaspoon orange juice

2 tablespoons milk

2 tablespoons mineral water

Throw the yogurt, lemon juice, lime juice, grapefruit juice, and orange juice into a small bowl. I prefer freshly squeezed, if possible. Mix well with a spoon and apply to the face for 10 minutes. Rinse off with lukewarm tap water followed by mineral water on a cotton ball. Now top it off by splashing on the milk and rinsing with tap water. Your skin will love it!

The Double Antioxidant

Grapes are all the rage these days owing to their antioxidants and restorative properties. This antioxidant toner is brilliant for women of all ages, but especially for those in their thirties trying to prevent sun damage and wrinkles. The combination of wine and grapes delivers two powerful antioxidants.

INGREDIENTS

    2 tablespoons wine

    10 grapes

Total time:
3 minutes

Blend the wine and grapes in a blender for 1 minute and make sure the grape skins are crushed up. Let the mixture sit on the face a couple of minutes before rinsing off. This is a good toner to put on after your cleanser and before you apply lotion.

✳ WEAR SUNSCREEN! ✳

*A*lso keep in mind, just as bottled water sitting in a hot car can be hazardous to your health, so can hot sunscreen. High temperatures can cause the ultraviolet-absorbing chemicals to degrade right in the bottle, despite the fact that sunscreen usually stays good for three years. So you may be applying nothing more than a cream to your skin that isn't protecting it from the harmful rays of the sun. Sunscreen should be kept at temperatures no warmer than about 75 degrees.

WELCOME ALL COUGARS!

These days, forty-year-old women are often mistaken for twenty-five-year-olds. Men in their twenties are hitting on my clients, and sometimes my clients take them up on it. Why not? Some of my most glamorous clients are in their forties. Listen, I have plenty of proud cougars who come in my office and I say, "Good for you!" Men have been getting away with it for years.

Now let's get to the tough stuff. Wrinkles, age spots, and a loss of elasticity are the biggest complaints of women in their forties. Suddenly the sun exposure from your teens and twenties is coming back to haunt you! Wrinkles may seem a bit more pronounced and your skin becomes more dehydrated. Then there's the problem of the skin becoming a little looser so the pores seem more visible.

Don't fret—these next recipes will do wonders for the forty-something crowd! First, let's tackle those ever-troubling patches of pigmentation. Here is a list of ways to combat brown spots and freckles:

Spot On

1. Lemon juice on freckles or age spots acts as a bleach. Apply nightly.

2. Alternate using olive oil and vitamin E after putting on lemon juice.

3. Onions don't just make you cry; they are also ideal for fading spots. Slice a red onion in half and rub on the area once a day.

4. Apply sour cream to clean skin and leave it on for fifteen minutes. Do this daily.

Spot Remover

My grandmother was obsessed with removing age spots. She became quite good at it over the years. All my clients who are over forty come in complaining about age spots! This next recipe can be applied to those stubborn spots on a daily basis. After a few months, you'll notice a huge difference.

INGREDIENTS

*Total time:
15–45 minutes*

    1 tablespoon hydrogen peroxide
    1 tablespoon whole milk

The hydrogen peroxide will make the milk foamy. Apply the mixture with foam to brown spots or freckles. Let it sit for 15 minutes and repeat the process three times (if you have the time).

Babushka's Beauty Tip:

I have a client who uses prescription bleaching cream to get rid of brown spots. She was having some good luck with it but noticed when she added this remedy, it made a dramatic difference.

Cream Cheese and Carrots

These days it's all about putting vitamin A in products. Here's a way to get it for under $2. The popular big brands charge over a hundred dollars for many products carrying vitamin A. Carrots have the highest content of beta carotene (vitamin A) of all vegetables. So enjoy some carrots and cream cheese. Put it on your bagel for breakfast, too! (Not the carrots, just the cream cheese.) I have a client who swears by this recipe and thinks it also does wonders on blackheads. My grandmother used to make this recipe with buttermilk, but I love the texture of the cream cheese.

INGREDIENTS

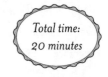

Total time:
20 minutes

   3 tablespoons cooked carrots

   3 tablespoons cream cheese

Throw the cooked carrots and cream cheese in the blender for 1 minute on high. Apply the creamy mixture to the face and neck for 15 minutes. Wash off with lukewarm water and pat dry.

Cocoa Mask

This dark chocolate mask will nourish the skin — and it's quite tasty! Of course, chocolate is high in antioxidants. Now that you know some of the benefits of chocolate, not only can you be guilt-free while eating it, but you can prepare an excellent chocolate face mask recipe to help preserve your skin's youthful look.

INGREDIENTS

Total time:
20 minutes

   ⅓ cup cocoa

   ¼ cup honey

    2 tablespoons sour cream

    3 teaspoons oatmeal powder

    1 teaspoon fresh orange juice

Put the ingredients in a blender on high until the mixture is smooth. Apply on the face, gently massaging it in. The oatmeal will exfoliate the skin. Leave the mask on for 15 minutes and rinse with lukewarm water.

MOVING TOWARD—
FIFTIES, SIXTIES,
SEVENTIES . . .

The skin game isn't over! Although women are aging better than ever, it's still important to realize that lower estrogen levels and gravity are working against us. However, if you know the facts about aging, there are plenty of ways to fight it. The face needs moisture. Think of it as a lawn constantly needing water.

I just met a woman who came in for a facial and I assumed she was forty-five. She was sixty-two! I've never seen anything like it. She definitely hadn't had any surgery. I asked, "How do you look so good?" She replied, "I do everything, but in moderation." She eats a little chocolate every day, has a glass of wine each night, and still eats meat. But she does wear sunscreen and exfoliates regularly. I would chalk some of it up to good genes as well.

Here are some tips for aging gracefully:

1. Exfoliate regularly to banish dry flakes that may collect makeup.

2. Use a powerful antioxidant moisturizer to stave off the signs of aging and prevent further damage.

3. Perform regular facials to maintain your complexion.

4. Apply an eye cream daily to fend off wrinkles and fine lines.

5. Use moisturizing foundation, which is the cornerstone of looking good. Dry skin gives away your age.

Do you know what my babushka did to plump up her face every morning and night? She'd take distilled water, freeze it, and then put it in the refrigerator overnight. In the morning, she'd splash that cold water on her face followed by hot water she boiled up. She would repeat this a few times. Now I don't always recommend this, but in a crunch it will plump up your face—especially if you're really tired.

Even when she was in her seventies, people would comment on my babushka's skin. She religiously used these masks. With flawless skin, she would often say, "The face is like the body—one *must* keep it looking firm and healthy." Despite having little money, my grandmother managed to prove beauty didn't come from a bottle or a syringe, but rather from nature. These recipes truly shaved twenty years off her appearance. Although she wasn't a terribly vain woman, she sure loved the compliments!

My grandmother was always looking for ways to keep her skin moist. She would use olive oil daily. There's nothing better for dry skin. Just keep it in your shower and apply it all over the body and face and rinse with water. A moisturizing film will remain. In women, after menopause, decreased estrogen levels mean that skin loses a bit of its plumpness and tone, and it may feel very dry, so moisturizing is key.

Pomegranate Punch

We all know how brilliant pomegranates are for the skin and body! They are a great antioxidant! This next recipe will do wonders to add moisture to the skin. My babushka always loved using cottage cheese in her recipes. As she got into her fifties and sixties, she used it on her own skin daily. Check this next recipe out . . .

Total time:
20 minutes

INGREDIENTS

    2 tablespoons pomegranate seeds

    2 tablespoons cottage cheese

    1 tablespoon buttermilk

Throw all the ingredients in a blender and blend them on high for 2 minutes. The mixture should resemble a smoothie. Place the mask all over your face and leave it on for 15 minutes. Rinse with lukewarm water.

Honey, Honey

There is nothing better for putting moisture back in the skin than honey. This recipe will leave your skin moist and glowing! Coconut oil is also great for dry skin and for people with eczema. When our skin is dry, it soaks up these natural products and gives the face a more youthful look. I always say soak in it and then glow in it!

INGREDIENTS

> 1 egg
>
> ½ cup coconut oil
>
> 1 tablespoon honey
>
> 2 tablespoons mineral water (for later)

Total time: 15 minutes

Mix the egg in a bowl. Then add the coconut oil and honey until the mixture has a smooth consistency. Apply on the skin for 5–10 minutes. Wash off with lukewarm water followed by mineral water. Since you'll have some extra mixture left over, add ¼ teaspoon of vodka to preserve the mask and store in the refrigerator.

Summer Sour Cream

During the summer you may need this recipe. My grandmother had one friend come to the house regularly. The woman had a number of brown spots on her face. By using a heavy mask with milk, sour cream, and honey, we watched those spots fade over time. (By "time," I don't mean weeks, but a few months.) Most of all, this recipe pumps up the skin and makes it feel silky smooth. Once I came to the States, I substituted cottage cheese for milk and found it worked a little better.

INGREDIENTS

> I teaspoon cottage cheese
>
> I teaspoon sour cream
>
> I teaspoon honey

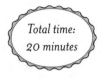

Total time:
20 minutes

Put all the ingredients in a blender and mix until they resemble a smoothie. Apply to the skin before bed and leave on for 10 minutes. Wash off with warm tap water. This is a fantastic recipe but it has to be done every night in order to see results. This cottage cheese soufflé will last one week in the fridge (unless you use ¼ teaspoon of the vodka-servative).

Cucumber Delight

If you want good skin, then cucumber is one way to get it! It creates skin that is both soft and smooth. Because of its soothing effect, a cucumber can literally work magic on the entire face. Putting some kind of cucumber mask on your face every few days can transform your skin.

INGREDIENTS

> 2 tablespoons instant nonfat
>
>   dry milk
>
> ½ peeled cucumber
>
> I tablespoon buttermilk

Total time:
25 minutes

Put all the ingredients into a blender and mix until smooth. Apply to your face, avoiding the eyes. Leave on for 15–20 minutes, and then rinse off with lukewarm water.

Babushka's Beauty Tip:

There is something very calming in cucumber. It's the first thing to apply to swollen eyes and it can really revitalize the skin within minutes. I'm always surprised by the power of this veggie!

Chapter Thirteen

One-Ingredient Wonders!

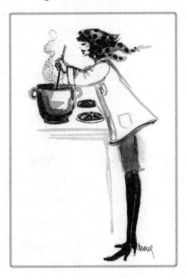

This is one of my favorite chapters because it's one ingredient and you're out the door! In this crazy world where multitasking has become a badge of honor, one-ingredient wonders seem perfect for those weeks when you're on the go and just, well, exhausted. You can literally grab one ingredient and get glamour-to-go.

Back in the Ukraine, my grandmother would make rather elaborate concoctions all day long for other people. Once in a while, after putting in twelve hours of work, she'd want to pamper the family, too. But after a long day, the idea of firing up the stove again seemed too overwhelming. That's when she'd turn to our one-ingredient wonders.

When I first arrived in the United States, I'd apply these one-ingredient wonders but wouldn't tell women what the product was in fear of their reaction. "You just put an orange on my face?" I thought they'd scream. But as each satisfied customer left the salon, my confidence grew. I finally relented and blurted out the truth. Their reactions were better than I'd ever expected. Clients were shocked and pleasantly surprised by the simplicity of it all.

The positive feedback I received upon revealing my "secret" ingredients is one of the reasons I decided to write this book. Clients really didn't care about all the fancy packaging, just if a beauty treatment worked. Because all my natural products are so effective, women all over Los Angeles began embracing these one-ingredient remedies—even dubbing them "the wonders of the beauty world."

You'll be surprised by the results in this chapter. Before telling you how to use each ingredient, I'll explain what makes it so special. There is no prep work and you'll never have to make last-minute spa appointments again! After learning about these quick fixes, you'll wonder why you spent so much money on those department store brands.

But let me just offer up one little warning by saying that many of the recipes in this chapter can be quite messy. Rubbing a tomato on your face isn't pretty, but your skin will be once you wash it off. Trust me, the results will outweigh the mess.

Orange Infusion

My babushka loved putting oranges directly on the skin. We did it whenever there were oranges in the house. A slice of orange is better than vitamin C serum for the face. Not just because it's a fraction of the price but because it's also the best way to get vitamin C. In this case, you're going straight to the source. Sure you can pay a couple hundred dollars for a fancy bottle, but who knows how diluted it is before it finally reaches your skin?

Peel a whole orange, then take a slice of the orange, cut off the very top, squeeze it, and the pulp will come out. Rub it 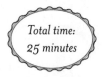 all over the face. You'll have pulp on the face but allow your skin to eat it up. Keep it on for 20 minutes. There's strong support behind vitamin C research and how it can reverse the aging process. C helps stimulate collagen, decreases wrinkles, and creates a gorgeous glow!

Total time: 25 minutes

Strawberry Hill

They're tasty and they're amazing for the skin! Strawberries will do wonders for your complexion. They have tons of vitamin C, which is the great skin restorer because it helps produce the big C—collagen— exactly what we crave. People pay thousands of dollars to pump up their skin with bovine collagen and the human stuff. By putting strawberries on the face, we're doing it naturally. *Think of it as a natural injection without all the chemicals or pain.*

Place 5 strawberries in a blender and turn it on high for 1 minute or until smooth (you can also add a squeeze of fresh lemon if you'd like). Then cover the entire face and neck with the mask and let it stay on for 20 minutes. Wash it off with lukewarm water. For those with sensitive skin, it can be a bit strong. I often recommend following it up by soaking a cotton ball in a tablespoon of buttermilk and spreading it all over the face. Then wash off and apply moisturizer.

Babushka's Beauty Tip:

Feel free to substitute blueberries or black-berries instead of strawberries; they'll work just as well. I often put together a blueberry-strawberry mask. It can be a little messy, but it works! The antioxidants found in these fruits can protect the skin cells.

Garlic-to-Go

As I've said, my grandmother loved garlic. She didn't mind the smell. My babushka would often say, "It smells strong because it is strong!" She was right. Garlic wards off blackheads and acne and does wonders for the complexion. We can all put up with a strong odor in the name of beauty.

Garlic is also one of the best natural antibiotics. The highly odorous clove has strong medicinal powers for the skin. When I was a teenager, my grandmother constantly put garlic on my skin to get rid of acne and it really worked. Even as an adult, I immediately get out the garlic when a pimple starts to appear. I regularly put it on the sides of my nose to get rid of blackheads as well. I find eating garlic is also good for chasing away acne.

Cut open 1 clove of garlic and rub it on a pimple or an area where you want to get rid of blackheads. If you have a little extra time, squash a clove of garlic and boil a cup of hot water (it will take you only 10 minutes). Throw the entire smashed clove in the hot water. It becomes a garlic tonic and is a brilliant cleanser to use after washing your face (before applying night cream).

*Total time:
2 minutes*

Divine Avocado

Talk about a green goddess. Avocado can be used to treat a number of skin problems. It's a great antioxidant for the skin. Not to mention, it is fantastic for the hair as well—think of it as a deep conditioner. This is one of those fruits that can take care of the hair and the face since it is great for dry skin. Ancient Aztec, Mayan, and Incan beauties believed avocado could work magic on the skin. They were right. Avocado is rich in vitamins, minerals, and natural oils.

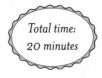

Mash up ¼ of a skinned avocado with a fork and blend until it's completely smooth. Run it through your fingertips

*Total time:
20 minutes*

and apply it all over the face for 15 minutes. Rinse off with lukewarm water. Once you're through with this mask, you'll be ready to take on the world. And don't forget, even if an avocado is overripe, you can still use it on your hair or face.

Babushka's Beauty Tip:

I often tell my clients if you're having a slow weekend, then do a double dose of avocado. You can simultaneously put this most nourishing fruit on your hair and face. Sure it's a little messy, but by the time the avocado is all off, you won't believe how luxurious you feel.

White Knight

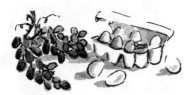

My grandmother loved eggs—she believed that no part of an egg should go to waste. In this next recipe you'll use the egg white, but save the yolks and shell for other recipes. Egg whites are fabulous as a tightening mask. In fact, when you apply them to your face, it will begin to feel a little uncomfortable after a few minutes as the egg white begins tightening the skin. Don't worry! Besides shrinking the pores, it gives your face an overall lift.

Crack 2 eggs and separate the egg whites. Beat the whites with a fork until they get foamy. Then spread them all over the face. It will take about 20 minutes for them to dry. Wash off the mask with cool water to reveal tighter pores and firmer, refreshed skin. (Don't forget to save the yolks in the refrigerator and use them in your hair—see Chapter 8. The shells should also be saved in the refrigerator, for recycling—see Chapter 14.)

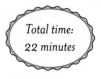

Total time: 22 minutes

OPTIONAL

Now take a tablespoon of buttermilk and a cotton ball and apply it all over the skin. Rinse off with lukewarm water after a few minutes.

Milk It!

I love goat's milk. It was once all the rage. That is, until cows bumped them aside and took the milk industry by storm. But goat's milk is making a comeback with research showing its many benefits. It's an ideal moisturizer and very calming for the skin since it has many nutrients to rejuvenate the face. Not to mention it's the ideal weapon in the fight against acne. I like using goat milk as a cleanser after a facial or in a bath. Those with eczema say it has magical properties. In ancient Egypt, Cleopatra was apparently a big fan and bathed in goat's milk. Although I think it's a great product, I'm not crazy about the smell.

Apply 1 tablespoon of goat's milk to the
skin after using any of the masks in
this book. Leave on for 5 minutes
and then wash off with lukewarm water.
You can use this milk as a daily cleanser.

Total time:
15 minutes

Yummy Yogurt

*I'm not surprised it's been called "the natural wrinkle remover from the
dairy case." I love yogurt. Strangely enough, it isn't as popular in the
Ukraine as it is in the United States.*

*Yogurt is the most popular fermented milk product in the United
States, but back in the Ukraine, it ranks among the lowest, although it
is starting to move up the food chain—and with good reason.*

*Since yogurt has antibacterial and antifungal properties, it's
excellent for cleansing the skin. In addition, the lactic acid in yogurt
soothes, softens, and tightens the skin. Remember, lactic acid is an
alpha hydroxy acid (AHA), which is brilliant for rejuvenating the skin.
Sometimes I'll even mix a teaspoon of ground orange peels in with a
couple tablespoons of yogurt to make an exfoliant that has a nice dose
of vitamin C. But as we all know, yogurt is pretty good with nothing on
it as well.*

Apply 2 tablespoons of plain yogurt to
your skin at any time. Spread it with a
cotton ball and leave on for 15 minutes.
Wash it off with lukewarm water and apply
a moisturizer.

Total time:
15 minutes

Babushka's Beauty Tip:

Yogurt is also good as a hair conditioner.
The active cultures in it can help fight off
dandruff. Add a little honey and throw it on
your hands and feet as well—it's an excellent moisturizer. Let's face it, yogurt is good
for everything from head to toe.

Pumpkin Paradise

*When you're carving those Halloween pumpkins, don't discard the
inside so quickly. The inside of a pumpkin is full of antioxidants and
vitamins. According to a report out of Duke University, when vitamin C
is applied directly to the skin, it can keep the skin's elastic fibers or collagen from breaking down (and pumpkin has a ton of vitamin C). Spa
and cosmetic companies are offering up an array of pumpkin facials
and pumpkin scrubs since this vitamin-rich veggie is good for everything
from exfoliating the skin to giving it a glow.*

Cut ¼ of a pumpkin (with the skin still
on) into small pieces. Remove the stringy
stuff along with the seeds. Place the pieces

*Total time:
50 minutes*

in a glass baking dish skin side up and fill it with 1 inch
of water. Cover it. Cook the pumpkin for 30 minutes at
350 degrees or until it gets soft. After taking the pumpkin out of the oven, let it cool. Cut the skin off the cooked
pumpkin and throw the rest into a food processor or
blender. Mix it on high for 2 minutes until it has a mashed

potato–like texture. Apply the mixture to the face for 15 minutes and rinse off with tap water.

Babushka's Beauty Tip:

I shouldn't be saying this, but I will. While I suggest fresh pumpkin, the canned stuff will do just fine. Plenty of my clients cheat on me with pumpkin in a can, but I always get them to confess. I'm a single mom and know how little time we all have in the day. I forgive them.

Honey Face Moisturizer

Honey is the ultimate moisturizer—it keeps the skin moist and dewy. There are a number of Hollywood beauties who swear by it! It's fantastic in helping the skin stay young and healthy. Honey has the ability to attract water, which helps plump the skin. It's great for sensitive skin since doctors often instruct patients with allergies to consume it to build up their immune system. Honey will minimize the appearance of facial wrinkles, and the antioxidants in honey will do wonders for the skin. My babushka believed every woman over forty should use honey on her face each and every day.

Total time: 25 minutes

Apply 1 tablespoon honey in a thin layer all over the skin and leave on for 20 minutes. (Make sure you wear a headband so it doesn't get all over your hair.) Wipe the honey off with a warm washcloth. Then apply a cleanser and follow your normal routine.

Babushka's Beauty Tip:

Honey is good for those pimples you couldn't help but perform surgery on—the ones we actually make worse. Put a drop of honey on your finger and place it on the pimple. Now put a Band-Aid over it (obviously best to do at night). Honey will aid in fighting off the bacteria, keep the skin sterile, and speed healing. It will work wonders by morning.

Babushka's Beauty Tip:

One high-profile actress rubs honey and salt all over her body on a regular basis to create a microdermabrasion effect while at the same time using the honey as a deep moisturizer.

Don't Hold the Mayo

It's surprising that I still love mayonnaise. It was literally something we consumed daily in the Ukraine. My babushka used it on everything! Mayo is the ultimate condiment. Women are also willing to put it in their hair to make it soft and shiny. What makes mayo so fattening is what makes it so healthy for the hair! It's basically made up of oil and egg yolks. The various fat-soluble nutrients in mayonnaise have a deep conditioning effect on the hair. Always use regular mayonnaise, none of the low-fat stuff. It simply won't work as well since lots of the fat is trimmed! This is one of those rare times we don't want reduced fat. *This is also another one of those times in which you'll save tons of money—mayo is one of the best (and least expensive) hair conditioners.*

Apply 2 tablespoons mayo to your hair. Don't put it too close to your roots or it could leave the hair very oily. I prefer

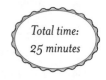

Total time: 25 minutes

putting it around the top and working down. Then draw it through to your ends until the hair is thoroughly coated. Pile the hair on top of your head. Put plastic wrap around the top of your head to hold the hair in place. Take a hot towel from the dryer and wrap it around your head over the plastic. The heat will aid with deep conditioning. Remove the towel and plastic wrap after about 10 minutes. Shampoo your hair as usual.

Babushka's Beauty Tip:

If the ends of your hair are damaged, do this once a week. If your scalp is naturally oily, you might want to add mayo only to the ends of your hair for weekly treatments.

Tomato Time

It took me a while to warm up to the idea of using tomatoes on the face since they're so messy. The thing is, they are very effective. This is the greatest remedy for oily skin. It tightens the pores and kills bacteria.

Tomatoes are very rich in vitamin C and perk up the skin! A number of cosmetic companies sell expensive creams and lotions with lycopene—an antioxidant found in tomatoes. They sell these products and tout how they get the lycopene directly from tomatoes. However, the products are also laced with a number of other ingredients and preservatives. Why do that when you can go straight to the source?

Cut a tomato in two, and rub one half on your face, working the pulp into the skin. I will admit this sounds

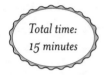

Total time:
15 minutes

(and is) a bit messy. Let it stay on your skin for 10 minutes. It's best to concentrate on areas where you want to attack blackheads and oil or reduce pores. Rinse with cool water (which is very crucial since the high acid content in tomato can make the skin a little sensitive).

OPTIONAL

Add two squeezes of lemon (for sensitive skin, substitute orange since it's less acidic).

Banana Babe

Bananas are ripe for creating good skin. They have certain enzymes that are ideal for skin care. Even the peel is good to rub on the skin. Because of their soothing properties, bananas are often used for reducing inflammation. Simply put, banana makes the skin soft and supple. This fabulous one-ingredient wonder will leave any type of skin feeling refreshed and pampered. But don't just relegate bananas to the face— they are ideal for conditioning the hair as well.

Mash ⅓ of a large banana until
smooth. Spread it all over the face and
leave on for about 15 minutes. The skin
will begin to feel tight. Rinse with
lukewarm water, then a small amount of cool water. Pat
your skin dry. This is a very refreshing mask and will
make your skin feel amazing!

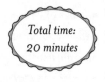

Total time:
20 minutes

Papaya, Please!

*Papaya is used in a number of trendy creams, lotions, shampoos,
scrubs, and salves. Even the skin of the papaya can be used to wash
one's face.*

*Papayas contain enzymes and antioxidants that battle prema-
ture aging. They do a fantastic job of exfoliating the skin as well. Did
you know that papaya has also become a leading ingredient in skin-
whitening products because it contains papain? Papain is a natural
enzyme that promotes skin renewal.*

*Apply it to the face and it diminishes wrinkles and nourishes the skin
with vitamin A, which accelerates the formation of new cells. In addition, it is rich in vitamin C, which is an antioxidant. Papaya plumps up
the skin and reduces the look of fine lines and wrinkles.*

Cut a papaya in half and remove the
seeds. Scoop out the flesh and place
it in a blender on high for 2 minutes.
Apply the mixture to the face and massage lightly. Leave it
on for 15 minutes and rinse with lukewarm water. Softly
pat the skin dry.

Total time:
20 minutes

Pineapple Express

Pineapple is perfect for the skin. It moisturizes and has those marvelous alpha hydroxy acids, as well as enzymes. These purify the skin while adding moisture and have the antiaging properties as well. Cosmetic companies often use pineapple in their products since it's a natural exfoliate.

Rub a piece of fresh pineapple all over your face. Leave on the skin for 10 minutes. You'll begin to feel the skin

Total time:
12 minutes

tighten. The pineapple juice will tighten the skin and the pores. It may make your face a little pink for a few minutes but you'll love the glow! Rinse with tap water. This is a treatment that's so easy it's a must to do weekly or even daily. Just applying a little pineapple to your skin will literally take minutes and the results will be dramatic. Don't let it get too close to your eyes.

Chapter Fourteen

Recycling Beauty

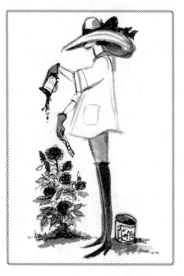

Without knowing it, my grandmother raised us all in what would (for the most part) be considered a green environment. We recycled everything from leftovers to eggshells. Before you toss anything out, read this chapter and you'll see how easy it is to recycle beauty. You've heard it over and over, but here it goes again: My grandmother didn't believe in waste. Leftovers rarely hit the trash—instead we often mixed up beauty concoctions from our breakfast, lunch, or dinner. After breakfast, eggshells were put to the side for a calcium lift while leftover bread brought a little bounce back to oily hair.

Bread was something we recycled constantly to take care of oily hair. However, the recipe—which involves throwing the bread into a boiling pot of water and then applying the wet (and disgusting) mush to the hair for 5 minutes—is quite messy. In fact, most of my clients think I'm nuts when I tell them about it.

My grandmother was always brewing up bread, a mask, or a meal. Using beets, potatoes, onions, and a variety of other items, she'd whip up a traditional Russian soup called borscht in a large vat on an open fire. Anything she didn't use would turn into leftover glamour. Even an unfinished cognac, beer, or wine would be used in different recipes.

The peels of an orange didn't see the bottom of a trash bin, but rather the faces of my babushka's clients. Ironically, these leftovers are some of my most potent potions.

This is a chapter where you can save the environment and save money!

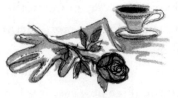

Flower Hour

Let's start with flowers! Why not recycle them when they begin to wilt? Flowers are so wonderful and deserve a second life. When your partner buys you a dozen roses, there's no need to throw them out after a week.

Simply take off the wilted petals and bathe in them! You won't believe how luxurious it feels! Then you can enjoy those lovely roses one more time.

INGREDIENTS

1–2 cups rose petals

½ cup coconut milk

¼ cup olive oil

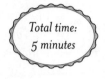

Total time: 5 minutes

Get a warm bath going and throw in the rose petals. Toss in the coconut milk and olive oil. Jump right in!

Coffee Sugar Scrub

Millions of Americans drink coffee every day. What happens to those leftover grounds? They sit in the coffeemaker for hours and then it's off to the trash with them! Don't waste them. Here's a great recipe that combines the leftover grounds with brown sugar. Not only is it amazing, but it produces an incredible aroma! My clients love this scrub since they feel it does wonders to the body and gives the skin a slight golden color.

INGREDIENTS

¼ cup sweet almond oil

1 teaspoon vanilla extract

1 cup granulated brown sugar

½ cup fresh coffee grounds

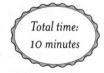

Total time: 10 minutes

In a medium glass bowl, combine all the ingredients and mix them together well with a spoon. You now have the ultimate body scrub! I suggest preparing this recipe when the coffee grounds are still warm since it makes the scrub feel a little more luxurious when it's applied.

✳ GIVE BRUNETTES A BOOST ✳

*T*his is a good tip that may sound a little crazy, but coffee grounds can help your hair, especially if you're a brunette! Not only will coffee grounds enhance the color of brown and black hair, but they also give your hair added shine. When you're in the shower, simply rub the used coffee grounds into your scalp and throughout the hair. Let it sit for 10 minutes and shampoo and condition your hair.

✳ COFFEE GROUNDS ✳

*a*s someone who can't live without her morning coffee, I'm proud to put those coffee grounds to use in ways beyond beauty.

1. **Make homemade tattoos (temporary).** Henna and coffee grounds can act as a sort of natural dye.

2. **Use coffee grounds to repel ants.** Try making a circle of old coffee grounds around an anthill.

3. **Keep felines from using your yard as a litter box.** Simply spread used coffee grounds and orange peels throughout the targeted areas.

4. **Freeze out odor.** Place a bowl of used coffee grounds in the freezer (or refrigerator) to remove bad odors.

5. **Rub coffee grounds on your hands to get rid of odors.** They work well on onions and garlic!

(cont.)

✳ COFFEE GROUNDS (CONT.) ✳

6. **Make a used coffee grounds sachet.** Fill old nylons with used coffee grounds. Now put them in your closets or place inside drawers to absorb odors. You can add a touch of vanilla if you'd like.

7. **Prepare a flea powder for pets.** After you give your dog or cat a bath (I know kitties hate baths), rub coffee grounds all over their fur. The coffee grounds should deter those dreaded fleas.

Eggshells and Buttermilk

We can even recycle eggshells. This high-calcium mask will change the texture of your skin! Who knew eggshell could be so irresistible? Just make sure the shells are blended very well because they can be very sharp if not. This is truly one of the most luxurious masks for the skin.

INGREDIENTS

3 eggshells

1 tablespoon buttermilk

2 tablespoons mineral water (for later)

Total time: 25 minutes

Pour all the ingredients into a blender and put it on high for 2 minutes. If you happen to have one of those small fast-touch coffee grinders, throw the ingredients inside and turn it on for a minute or two. Remember these shells need to be in a powder form. Spread the mask on your face and leave on for 15 minutes. Rinse with cool tap water followed by mineral water.

> ## Babushka's Beauty Tip:
>
> Talk about egg on the face! My clients over forty love this mask. It's an instant calcium infusion. The Eggshells and Buttermilk mask is one of the most powerful masks for women who are facing dry skin problems.

Teatime

Let me start by saying that this isn't a complicated recipe but there is a little work involved. If you're having some girlfriends over, this is a nice way to recycle and enjoy a little tea. Offer your friends a choice of chamomile or green tea. Then reuse the tea bags to take away puffiness and dark circles under the eyes.

INGREDIENTS

Total time: 20 minutes

2 chamomile tea bags

1 teaspoon honey

2 green tea bags

Place the tea bags in separate boiling cups of water and add a dash of honey to each. Let the tea bags sit for 5 minutes and throw them in the refrigerator until the bags are no longer hot, but still a little warm. First, put the chamomile compresses on the eyes for 3 minutes, then trade them for the green tea. It sounds like a hassle but your eyes will look beautiful and refreshed!

THE POTENCY OF
THE PEELS

No need to discard the peels of many of your favorite fruits and vegetables. These can be recycled in some of the most incredible ways:

Grapefruit Delight

Don't throw away the empty half from your morning grapefruit either. It can keep your elbows soft and youthful looking. You know the area where the skin just sort of loosely hangs and at times can seem to get a bit darker. This will lighten up the skin while at the same time keeping it soft and supple. Just let your elbows rest inside the two halves of the grapefruit while you watch TV. (I know it sounds a bit insane but it's honestly easier than cutting up the grapefruit skin.) However, you can cut it up into smaller pieces and just rub the peel on your elbows if you prefer.

Banana Peels Aren't Funny—They're Serious Beauty Business!

Rubbing a banana peel on your skin is amazing as well! The peel contains potassium and lutein, which is an antioxidant. It may sound a bit disgusting but rubbing the peel on your face can be quite incredible. Banana peel is also known to be good for making pimples disappear after a couple uses.

Precious Pumpkin

Don't ever get rid of the pumpkin rind. There are some doctors who claim rubbing it all over the face will dramatically improve your skin texture. Orange squash is said to contain several ingredients that help the skin look and feel younger. One plastic surgeon is so taken with pumpkin rind he even offers a special peel to his patients. He claims wrinkles become softer and it produces an amazing glow. It does!

Orange Alert

Orange peel absorbs the oils from open pores in your skin, thereby helping reduce the greasy shine on the face caused by excess oil. It also helps to pick up dead and dry skin cells from the surface, making the face look brighter and cleaner. Simply rub the white part of the skin all over the face.

Pining for Papaya

The skin of the ripe papaya can be thrown in the fridge and used to invigorate the face. Simply apply the fleshy side of a green papaya skin all over the face. It helps eliminate dead skin and makes your skin feel great. It's brilliant!

BEER ADDS BODY

Beer Shampoo and Conditioner

Most women will spend close to $50 to add a little bounce to their mane. Beer is the less expensive alternative. So next time you need a little oomph, grab that leftover beer—it's the ultimate conditioner for hair. It will add both body and shine. Below are two of my favorite recipes. (The beer should be flat.) There is a ton of protein in beer's malt and hops!

INGREDIENTS

> 1 tablespoon of your favorite
> shampoo
> 1 teaspoon flat beer
> 1 egg yolk

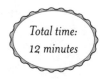

*Total time:
12 minutes*

Mix the ingredients together, then use it as your shampoo. Leave on 5–10 minutes, then rinse well. Now put a little more beer on your hair in the shower for the ultimate in double conditioning. Your hair will be so full and shiny!

Beer Body

This recipe will add body and shine to your mane!

INGREDIENTS

> 1 cup flat beer
> 1 teaspoon jojoba oil

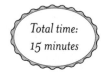

*Total time:
15 minutes*

In a small bowl, mix the two ingredients together. After shampooing, apply this mixture to towel-dried hair, carefully working it through the entire head. Leave the beer and oil concoction on for 10 minutes. Rinse with lukewarm water.

Babushka's Beauty Tip:

Some of Hollywood's greatest beauties pour beer in their hair regularly to make it shiny. These are women who can afford the best of the best and they still prefer beer.

Chapter Fifteen

Babushka's Words of Wisdom

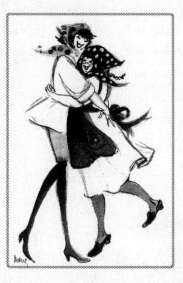

Thank you for allowing me to share my babushka's recipes. I am honored. From beer to bananas to bathing in bubbles, I am so excited for you to begin trying the different recipes. My family was convinced that once I came to the States, I'd stop brewing up beauty. At first, the thought of buying beauty products in a department store was appealing because of the packaging, promotion, and promises. But I found empty promises in beautiful packaging. And I began to miss the process of making it myself.

As I said in the first chapter, I didn't believe there was a market for my babushka's recipes, but now I realize why people are embracing them with such gusto. There is a certain satisfaction that comes from making your own products at home and discovering they actually work better! I am thrilled to bring these recipes to new generations. My grandmother would be proud!

Every morning as I pour a cup of coffee and rub olive oil all over my face, I think of my babushka. She was always slathering her face in oil and sipping black tea or coffee.

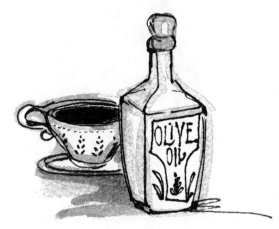

She would be proud to know I am using olive oil on a daily basis. As I said before, it was an expensive commodity back then so we had to use sunflower oil. My babushka was ahead of her time, not just in making preservative-free products, but in looking at women the way she did. She believed that women possessed great power. Much more than they even knew. My babushka was born in 1927 and was way ahead of her time. She truly loved creating different concoctions and making women smile.

She was never shy to express her opinion and was an extremely wise woman. Her words of wisdom are on the next page. I hope you enjoy reading them!

Babushka's Words of Wisdom

✳ Always keep a healthy mind and body—a woman must take care of herself! One must try to stay healthy both mentally and physically because if the mind suffers, eventually the body will, too.

✳ Age is only a number—instead of becoming obsessed with staying young, one should embrace one's age, look one's best, and live life with a youthful spirit.

✳ In relationships, women are always in control—because women are naturally more evolved than men, it's their responsibility to be the matriarchs and keep the family together.

✳ Never underestimate the power of friendship—girlfriends should always support and be loyal to one another. And remember there's nothing better than bonding with women over spa treatments and a little vodka.

✳ Never spoil your children—children are the greatest gift of all. Love them unconditionally, but spoil them and they'll live with you for life.

✳ The soul of a home should always be the kitchen—there is nothing more comforting than to enter a home alive with people cooking together in the kitchen and filling the air with delicious aromas.

✳ True happiness is helping others—giving to others is always more gratifying than receiving.

✳ Don't waste—there is no reason to waste anything. Not only does it burn money but it also wastes our world's precious resources. Remember almost everything has a dual purpose and can be reused in one way or another.

✳ Find a mate who brings out the best in you—be with someone who makes you happy, and remember, you can't truly love another until you love yourself first.

✳ Find your passion in life—once you discover what you are passionate about, success and happiness will follow.

So get a glass of wine and mix up a mask. *Na zdorovie!* Here's to my babushka!

Index

Index

Index

About the Authors

~~~~~~~~~~~~~~~~~~~~~~~~~~~

RAISA RUDER

As a child in the Ukraine, Raisa Ruder would whip up natural recipes with her grandmother and marvel at the results they'd produce. After noticing all the preservatives in products in America, she decided to introduce her recipes to the States and has quickly become the go-to girl in Hollywood.

On any given day, Raisa Ruder's Beverly Hills salon reveals the ecofriendly glamour so sought out in Tinseltown today. Wrapped in a chic white organic cotton apron, she throws together ingredients with the confidence and passion reminiscent of Julia Child. Only in this case, Ruder is cooking up soufflés for the skin, rather than the dinner table.

SUSAN CAMPOS

Susan Campos met Raisa Ruder when she was writing a story about green beauty. She immediately loved Raya's beauty regime, and a few years later they decided to do a book together.

Susan worked as an anchor/reporter in a number of television markets throughout the United States. She then joined NBC News, where she anchored the national weekend edition of *The Today Show*, reported for NBC, and hosted a number of entertainment shows for MSNBC.

She now lives in Los Angeles with her son and writes trend stories for *The New York Times, The Huffington Post*, as well as a number of other publications. Susan also has a blog called Beauty Undercover.